49 WAYS TO EAT
YOURSELF WELL

MARTINA WATTS MSC NUT MED

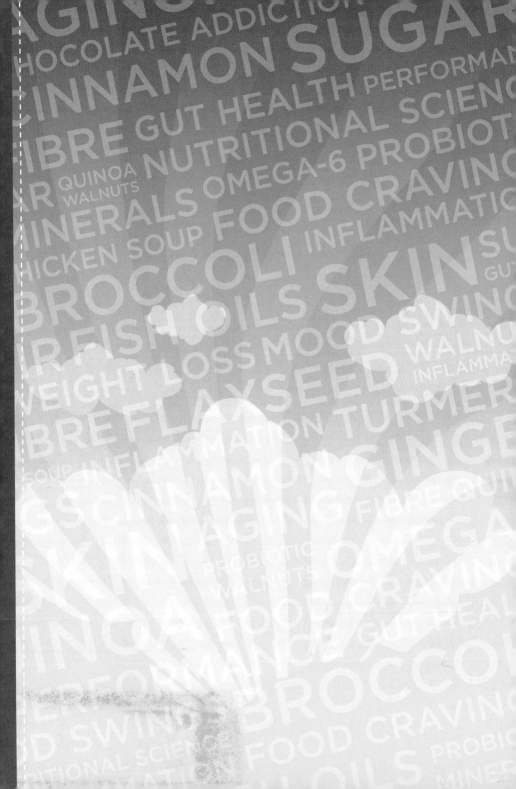

49 WAYS TO
EAT
YOURSELF WELL

Nutritional science one bite at a time

MARTINA WATTS MSC NUT MED

First published in Great Britain in 2013 by Step Beach Press Ltd, Brighton

Copyright © Martina Watts

The right of Martina Watts to be identified as the author of the work has been asserted in accordance with the Copyright, Designs and Patents Act 1988.

The series copyright, establishing the format and presentation of this material, is held by Step Beach Press.

A CIP catalogue record for this title is available from the British Library.

ISBN: 978 1 908779 06 9

Photographs by www.dreamstime.com, www.depositphotos.com and www.flickr.com

Series editor Jan Alcoe

Edited by Jo Hathaway

Typeset in Brighton, UK by Keren Turner at Katch Creative

Cover design by Keren Turner at Katch Creative

Printed and bound by Star Standard Industries, Singapore

Step Beach Press Ltd, 28 Osborne Villas, Hove, East Sussex BN3 2RE

www.stepbeachpress.co.uk

For my sons, Joe and Dion, my extraordinary daily reminders that I need to eat well to be well.

Acknowledgements

In recognition of all who work to achieve quality nutrition: cooks and food-growers everywhere, nutritionists, writers and scientists past, present and future. You are inspirational.

49 Ways to Well-being Series

If you have selected this book, you may be looking for practical ways of improving your well-being. If you are a health and well-being practitioner or therapist, you may be helping your clients to improve theirs by encouraging them to practise some of the approaches it is based on. Well-being is a subjective state of 'feeling good' which has physical, mental, emotional and even spiritual dimensions.

Because these dimensions overlap and interact, it is possible to improve well-being by making positive changes in any one of them. For example, taking up regular exercise (a focus on physical well-being) may improve concentration (mental well-being), happiness (emotional well-being) and sense of purpose (spiritual well-being). This series of well-being books is designed to provide a variety of routes to recovering, sustaining, protecting and enhancing well-being, depending on your interests and motivations. While some emphasise psychological techniques, others are based on physical movement, nutrition, journaling and many other approaches.

Each book in the series provides 49 practical ways of improving well-being, based on a particular therapeutic approach and written by an expert in that field. Based on tried and tested approaches, each title offers the user a rich source of tools for well-being. Some of these can be used effectively for improving general resilience; others are particularly helpful for specific problems or issues you may be dealing with, for example, recovering from illness, improving relaxation and sleep, or boosting motivation and self-confidence.

Enjoy dipping into any *49 Ways* book and selecting ones which catch your interest or help you to meet a need at a particular time. We have deliberately included many different ideas for practice, knowing that some will be more appropriate at different times, in different situations and with different individuals. You may find certain approaches so helpful or enjoyable that you build them into everyday living, as part of your own well-being strategy.

Having explored one book, you may be interested in using some of the other titles to add to your well-being 'toolbox', learning how to approach your well-being via a number of different therapeutic routes.

For more information about the series, including current and forthcoming titles, visit **www.stepbeachpress.co.uk/well-being**

CONTENTS

1 2 3 4 5 6 7 8

9 10 11 12 13 14

15 16 17 18 19

20 21 22 23 24

25 26 27 28 29

30 31 32 33 34

35 36 37 38 39

40 41 42 43 44

45 46 47 48 49

INTRODUCTION

Welcome to *49 Ways to Eat Yourself Well*. This book features 49 proven methods to positively affect the way you think about food and your health. Study after study reaffirms the crucial role of a nutrient-rich diet (along with exercise) as one of the most powerful factors in maintaining health and fighting disease. It is all too easy to get stuck in a rut of daily routines and habits that undermine our health. With the advent of modern processed foods we have been persuaded to follow the path of convenience and 'least resistance' and this sort of diet tends to encourage a low performance mindset. It is surprisingly easy to forget how our food and beverage choices impact on our physical and mental performance. High performance that is sustainable rarely happens by chance, it happens by choice.

When I recommend nutritional strategies to my clients, they always want to know 'why' and how to put these recommendations into practice. This book is based on our conversations and the valuable and valued feedback I have received from them over many years, along with motivational and practical ideas based on the latest evidence in nutrition science and nutritional medicine.

I have also added interesting historical facts, folklore and remedies through the ages. Topics include managing inflammatory conditions; boosting immunity; stabilising blood sugar; improving digestion, and providing optimal nutrition for the brain. The emphasis is on increasing energy, vitality and resilience, thereby improving our ability not only to survive, but thrive at work or play in a rapidly changing environment.

The human diet has changed inestimably over centuries, especially since the domestication of animals and plants 10,000 years ago, and subsequently with the industrialisation of the human food-supply chain. Modern humans are genetically virtually identical to our hunter–gatherer ancestors, and so may be more attuned to our ancestral diet than the current standard fare. This is important because the new science of epigenetics suggests we are not simply born with genes that are pre-set for life; a number of genes may be affected by our environment and our diet choices.

Food contains many thousands of active components which can switch our genes on and off, or alter their function. We may therefore be able to protect ourselves and future generations by making appropriate changes to our diet and lifestyles. In isolation, of course, any type of food or nutrient is insufficient. We require the whole 'package', and this means eating, digesting, absorbing and utilising a variety of different compounds regularly so that it becomes a daily habit and pleasure, not a chore.

This book is not intended to be a cookbook advocating a particular diet. Although I confess to being partial to the old Mediterranean way of eating, in practice I have learned that we are all individuals, with our own particular preferences and requirements. My mantra is quality and economy of food, simplicity,

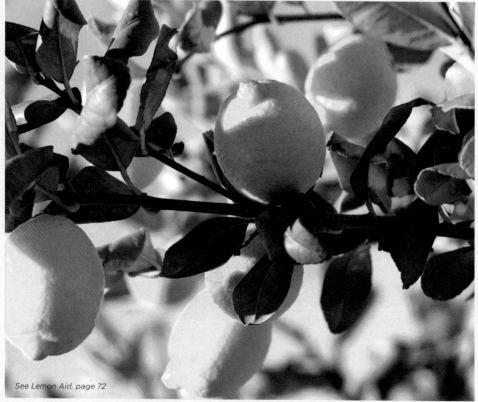

See Lemon Aid, page 72

easy digestibility and nutritional balance. Not everyone enjoys spending all their time in the kitchen, so I have incorporated recipes which are straightforward to assemble and take as little time as possible.

A good food blender is necessary for some recipes, and a juice extractor for the juices. If sensitive to dairy and gluten, you can easily use dairy and gluten-free alternatives that are available in any health store and many supermarkets. As my clients know, I am not a fan of concentrated doses of sweetness, such as refined or unrefined sugar, honey, molasses, golden syrup and so on. I recommend using dried or fresh fruit, a little honey or maple syrup whenever sweetness is required.

I have organised the *49 Ways* into three chapters:

- *Chapter 1*: Breakfast Ideas
- *Chapter 2*: Salads and Main Meals
- *Chapter 3*: Snacks and Desserts

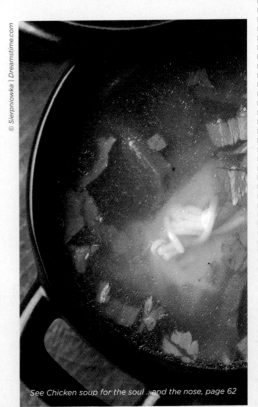
© Sierpniowka | Dreamstime.com

See Chicken soup for the soul ... and the nose, page 62

You will find note pages at the end of each chapter titled 'Recipe Variations and Substitutions'. Use them to record new recipes, or your own adaptations of the ones included. You can also make plans for how you can incorporate new foods into your diet.

You can dip in and out of the book as you wish – it need not be read sequentially as each 'Way' stands on its own merits and you can find benefit by choosing whichever one you like the look of. The more 'Ways' you choose, the more you increase your motivation to eat well. I suggest trying out one new food or recipe a week. Lunch and dinner recipes are interchangeable, as many people prefer to

eat a lighter meal in the evening. Some may even wish to eat soup for breakfast or use one of the snack options instead of a main meal. You may wonder why many delicious and healthy foods are not mentioned – this is simply because I only had 49 options!

GLOSSARY

The glossary lists and explains various nutritional terms that are mentioned in the book, and which we often hear or read but don't necessarily understand. It also lists specific nutrients mentioned throughout the book, and links them back to featured foods.

Any words that appear in the glossary have an asterisk next to them in the text, like this*.

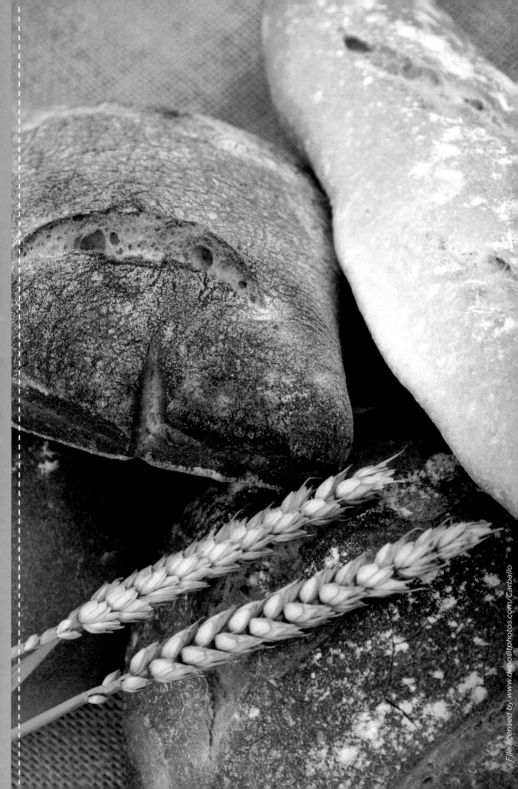

USEFUL RESOURCES

I have also included a list of useful websites and books for you to investigate.

THE 49 WAYS

Each numbered 'Way' provides a significant route to recovering, preserving or enhancing your well-being. It will usually include:

- underpinning theory, evidence or information on a particular food or food topic
- a handy **Tip** for incorporating the food into your regular diet
- a **Recipe** example featuring the particular food highlighted in that 'Way'
- **See Also** references to other featured foods
- key references so you can find out more about topics that interest you.

FINALLY...

This book is for anyone seeking to increase healthy habits for a more vital and energetic life and consistently improved mental and physical performance. It is also for those who feel tired all the time, overworked and overwhelmed, heading for a crisis or burnout, who want to be able to respond to challenges and cope with constant change and uncertainty. There is a wealth of tips and ideas for those who want to 'get ahead' and enjoy a richer, healthier quality of life.

NOTES ON THE RECIPES

Unless otherwise stated:

- 1 tsp = 5ml
- 1 tbsp = 15 ml
- 1 cup = 250 ml

Measurements are approximate, please feel free to experiment.

A NOTE OF WARNING

Food can be powerful medicine! The material in this book is intended for informational purposes and none of the suggestions are meant to be prescriptive. Always consult a nutritionally qualified healthcare professional for guidance in the use of foods, herbs or spices to prevent, manage or treat any health condition. If you suffer from a medical condition, please seek medical advice before changing your diet or introducing new ingredients. The recipes in this book have been begged, borrowed and collected from my lovely fellow nutritional therapists who are always willing to share, and my wonderful family, friends and clients. I am hugely indebted to them all.

1 2 3 4 5 6 7 8
9 10 11 12 13 14
15 16 17 18 19
20 21 22 23 24
25 26 27 28 29
30 31 32 33 34
35 36 37 38 39
40 41 42 43 44
45 46 47 48 49

Chapter 1

BREAKFAST IDEAS

Breaking your fast after hours of sleep can be tricky to get right. Breakfasts need to be nutrient-dense, invigorating and sustaining, without weighing you down. Smoothies are ideal for those in a hurry, refreshingly light and provide a host of antioxidants to support immunity. Nut loaves and muffins, prepared beforehand, also save time and are packed with protein and healthy fats to help prevent cravings for unhealthy snacks and energy dips throughout the morning.

The Bircher muesli is a great favourite in the summer, along with yoghurt and stewed cherries – both recipes are packed with nutrients, easy to digest and eat. On colder days, nothing is as warming as porridge made with oats, millet or other wholegrain cereals. Pancakes are comforting, too, with either sweet or savoury toppings, and are popular at weekends. Eggs provide a useful and economical source of protein, but if you fancy an alternative to boiling, poaching or scrambling, try a delicious tortilla.

All recipes can be made without gluten or dairy (milk alternatives such as soya, coconut, rice and nut milks, and gluten-free flour and oats are now widely available in supermarkets and health stores).

WAY 1

A taste of cherry

**Whoever said 'Life is a bowl of cherries...'
had the right idea, nutritionally speaking**.

Sometimes sweet and sometimes sour, cherries
can lay claim to be 'superfruits', so rich are
they in the naturally-occurring phytonutrients*
increasingly associated with health benefits.
The juicy fruit has evidently been enjoyed since
prehistoric times and one fondly imagines even
Stone Age children happily engaged in cherry
stone spitting competitions. Currently, there
are more than a thousand varieties of cherry
trees worldwide.

Cherries are a rich source of vitamin* C,
beta-carotene*, potassium*, iron, plant
melatonin* and natural plant pigments
such as the anthocyanins* and carotenoids*.
Such a potent cocktail of compounds is
likely to have significant antioxidant* and
anti-inflammatory effects. Indigenous people
such as the Native Americans, who had an
instinctive understanding of the healing
properties of plant foods, certainly thought
so. They prepared teas and infusions from
the bark and leaves of the cherry tree to
relieve pain and diarrhoea, and to treat
coughs, colds and sore throats.

Research suggests that consuming
antioxidant-rich fruit and vegetables triggers
cellular responses in our bodies that increase
our own antioxidant defence mechanisms,
thereby slowing down oxidative processes
and free radical damage that contribute to
ageing and disease (1).

There is particular scientific and commercial
interest in the antioxidant capacity of a tart
variety of cherries grown primarily in North
America, called Montmorency cherries
(Prunus cerasus).

Montmorency cherries are one of the richest
sources of anthocyanins, the plant pigments
which provide cherries with their deep red
colour. Anthocyanins are thought to be
beneficial in the management and prevention
of inflammatory diseases, as they block
enzymes* produced in the body that are
involved in causing inflammation. Reducing
chronic inflammation may offer protection
against heart disease and stroke, ease arthritic
pain, reduce the risk of insulin resistance and
diabetes, improve cognitive function and
speed muscle recovery in athletes after
intense exercise (2). Daily consumption of
these tart cherries has also been found to
lower blood levels of uric acid, relieving the
discomfort of gout.

Montmorency cherries are one of the
few known dietary sources of melatonin.
Produced by humans in the pineal gland*
in the brain, melatonin is not only a potent
antioxidant, but acts as a hormone. It is
involved in regulating our circadian rhythms*
and natural sleep patterns (3). As around a
third of adults in Western countries experience
difficulties sleeping (4), independent
studies are required to discover whether
the consumption of Montmorency cherries
increases melatonin levels in the blood and
might therefore improve sleep.

SEE ALSO
- **WAY 2: Almonds, the all-rounders**
  (page 20)
- **WAY 44: Honey, honey** (page 116)

Stewed Summer Cherries

An inspired way to serve cherries and a wonderfully healthy
start to your day when combined with yoghurt or porridge.

Ingredients

1 cup cherries, pitted and quartered
1 tbsp balsamic vinegar
2 tbsp honey
Live yoghurt (or soya yoghurt)
1 tsp chopped nuts

Serves 2

Method

1. In a small saucepan, stir together the honey and vinegar. Add cherries and mix well.

2. Place over medium-high heat. Bring to a boil and then simmer gently for 8–10 minutes, leaving uncovered and stirring occasionally. Remove from heat.

3. Serve cherries warm with vanilla ice-cream for dessert, or allow to cool and enjoy with live yoghurt for breakfast. Sprinkle with chopped nuts.

Tip: Sweet cherries are a great snack food and lunchbox treat. Tart cherries, including Montmorency cherries, are dried, canned for use in pies or made into juice concentrate.

WAY 2

Almonds, the all-rounders

Nuts, including wild almonds and acorns were already a major part of the human diet 780,000 years ago, during the Pleistocene period.

They come perfectly packaged to preserve their highly nutritious content, and our hunter–gatherer ancestors developed a variety of tools such as pitted hammers and anvils to crack them open (5).

Nuts are a valuable addition to most diets. Studies have consistently shown an association between regular nut consumption and a reduced risk of coronary heart disease. Long-term nut consumption is also linked to lower body weight and lower weight gain, despite their reputation of being high in fat. They encourage weight loss by improving blood sugar control, boosting satiety and suppressing hunger for longer.

Walnuts are particularly nutritious and contain higher amounts of antioxidants than almonds, hazelnuts, Brazil nuts, cashews, macadamias and pecans. Walnuts also supply a significant amount of ALA, the plant-based source of omega-3* fatty acids*. When exposed to heat, light and air, these polyunsaturated fats* oxidize quickly, so it is best to store shelled walnuts in an airtight container in the fridge (for up to 6 months) or freezer (for up to 1 year) to ensure freshness. In-shell walnuts will remain fresh for several months when stored in a cool, dry place.

My favourite nut is the almond, a stone fruit related to cherries, plums and peaches and grown primarily in Southern Europe and California. The Spanish believe that eating five almonds a day keeps them healthy, and there is no doubt that these nuts are exceptionally nutritious. Almonds are a rich source of vitamins E and B2, magnesium*, manganese*, plant sterols*, fibre, protein and monounsaturated fatty acids. They are also one of nature's best sources of the amino acid* tryptophan* which the body converts into the 'feelgood' brain chemical serotonin*.

Research suggests that eating almonds regularly is cardioprotective as they reduce low-density lipoprotein* (LDL) cholesterol in both healthy individuals and those with high cholesterol and diabetes (6, 7). They are excellent for digestion as the fibrous skin of almonds has a prebiotic effect. Prebiotics* are non-digestible ingredients that provide a food source for the 'friendly' bacteria in our intestines and encourage their growth (8). Almonds can be ground into flour and used as a substitute for grain flour for those with digestive problems or grain intolerance. The flour is also highly beneficial for people suffering from diabetes as it contains little carbohydrate.

SEE ALSO
- **WAY 9: Most definitely go to work on an egg** (page 34)
- **WAY 42: Cinnamon, add some spice into your life** (page 112)
- **WAY 49: Versatile bananas for high energy** (page 126)

Tip: Soaking shelled almonds overnight, then draining and rinsing in fresh water helps to enhance their flavour and remove enzyme inhibitors*, making them easier to eat and digest.

Almond and Banana Loaf

There are endless versions of this famous low GI recipe, so do experiment with your own ideas. Instead of the banana you can use grated apple and/or carrots. Try adding grated ginger, dried fruit or berries. If you prefer a savoury variety, use grated courgette instead of the banana, omit the cinnamon and honey and add tomato puree, seeds, herbs, salt and pepper.

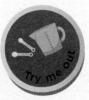

Ingredients

1 ¹/₂ cups almonds

1 cup pecan nuts

1 ripe banana

3-4 eggs

2 tbsp olive oil

1-2 tbsp honey
(or agave or maple syrup)

1 tsp baking powder

¹/₂ tsp cinnamon

(Recipe adapted from versions by Dr Natasha Campbell McBride and Christine Bailey – please see Useful Resources.)

Method

1. Grind the almonds and pecans to flour in a food processor or blender and pour into a large bowl (you can also use hazelnuts, cashews, pistachios or a mixture of these).

2. Combine with the baking powder and cinnamon.

3. Process all the other ingredients in a blender and add to the nut flour.

4. Mix well and pour the batter into a well-greased loaf pan. The mixture should be quite runny.

5. Bake at 160°C (325°F) for approximately 1 hour.

6. Cool before turning out and slicing. Delicious served with butter.

File licensed by www.depositphotos.com/Krysek

WAY 3
Apples are as good as they say, better in fact

Who can blame Eve for being unable to resist the luscious looks and sweet-smelling aroma of a fresh apple?

There are plenty of different ways to eat one. Some like it hot, some like it cold, some like it peeled and sliced. The best way, however, is to eat the whole fruit, core and all, until you are left with nothing but a little brown stalk. This has less to do with a 'waste not want not' philosophy and more to do with the fact that every part of an apple contains specific nutrients conducive to health.

Simply wash and go, for there is a much higher concentration of nutrients in the peel than in the flesh, and it seems almost sinful to throw away all those extra goodies. The peel contains the highest level of phenolic compounds* with corresponding antioxidant activity. These are health-promoting plant pigments and flavouring agents which may reduce the risk of chronic disease, including metabolic syndrome and Type 2 diabetes (9). Different apple varieties vary in their phenol compounds, and organic apples appear to have a higher total phenolic content than conventionally grown ones (10).

Another reason an apple or two a day keeps the doctor away is its high fibre content.

Fruit fibre has a variety of functions and one of the most important is to prevent constipation. Apples get the bowels moving – they are particularly high in the soluble fibre pectin which adds bulk and, as an added bonus, helps to eliminate excess cholesterol. Pectin also slows down digestion and reduces the speed of glucose absorption, making it an ideal snack for anyone wanting to stabilise blood sugar, although overly sweet apples should be avoided. Additionally, fibre such as pectin encourages the growth of 'friendly' bacteria in the digestive tract so they can keep your internal 'plumbing' in good working order (11).

The pioneering Swiss physician Maximilian Bircher-Benner (1867–1939) is rumoured to have cured himself of jaundice by eating raw apples, and went on to create the world-famous Bircher muesli. Grated or stewed, apples are a useful way of preventing dehydration in the elderly or the very young because of their high water content. They are also a good source of vitamin C, potassium, folic acid and other vitamins and minerals. Eating apples is an excellent way of clearing out your system if you need a quick detox. You may even reduce the symptoms of a hangover by eating a couple of apples on the morning after the night before!

SEE ALSO
- **WAY 2: Almonds, the all-rounders** (page 20)
- **WAY 4: Berry healthy for you** (page 24)
- **WAY 10: Oat cuisine** (page 36)

Tip: If stuck on a plane for a day, take a bag of apples with you and munch on these rather than the usual high-tech air food. Crunching on raw apples gives the jaws and gums a workout whilst simultaneously cleaning the teeth.

Creamy Bircher Muesli

The most famous muesli of all is also one of the tastiest and, if soaked overnight, easier to digest. Omit the yoghurt if sensitive to dairy.

Ingredients

$^{1}/_{2}$ cup porridge oats
A handful of almonds or pecans
A handful of blackberries, blueberries, dried cranberries or sultanas
Juice of $^{1}/_{2}$ lemon or orange
2–3 tbsp water
100ml live yoghurt
(or soya yoghurt)
1 grated apple
1 tsp honey if required
Cinnamon to taste

Method

1. Mix the oats with the nuts in a little added water and soak overnight.
2. In the morning, add the lemon juice, grated apple (with peel), berries and yoghurt.
3. Drizzle with honey and sprinkle cinnamon over the top.

Serves 1

Try me out

WAY 4

Berry healthy for you

One of the pleasures of late summer is picking juicy wild berries ready for freezing, jam-making or adding to apple pies.

Blackberries, raspberries, blueberries, bilberries, blackcurrants and strawberries are all highly nutritious and packed with essential nutrients. They are also low in calories and fat, and high in fibre*.

Berries are particularly rich in flavonoid compounds, including anthocyanins and flavonols*. These water-soluble pigments provide berries with their deep blue, red and purple colours, and their purpose is to protect them from sun damage. Flavonoids* are antioxidants, and regular consumption is believed to reduce the risk of degenerative disease.

Flavonoids from blueberries and strawberries may improve blood pressure (12). Even consuming relatively small amounts contributes to healthy blood flow and is associated with a reduced risk of death from heart disease (13). Berries also decrease the glucose response after a meal and may assist in the regulation of blood sugar. A recent study looked at the association of flavonoid subclasses and the risk of Type 2 diabetes. It was found that a higher consumption of flavonoids was linked to a lowered diabetes risk (14).

Blueberries are of particular interest as they have been found to improve mental performance. Animal studies show improvements in nerve cell communication, and there may even be some reversal of memory impairment (15). Along with cranberries, blueberries can be used for recurring urinary tract infections as they contain compounds that prevent bacteria from attaching to the delicate membranes of the bladder.

My favourite of all berries, however, is black elderberry, one of the best natural protective agents against cold and flu viruses. Unlike bacteria, a virus cannot replicate on its own and invades a healthy cell to produce new copies of itself. Black elderberry contains active components which prevent an invasion of the virus and stop it from multiplying. If you are lucky enough to have an elder tree in your garden, play hunter–gatherer and pick the tiny black-purple elderberries. Boil and strain them to make a soothing cordial for colds and coughs. If you are somewhat pressed for time, you can buy black elderberry in a liquid tincture from many health food stores or pharmacies. Berries are high in salicylates, natural aspirin-like compounds, and those who have low tolerance to salicylates may experience reactions.

SEE ALSO
- **WAY 2: Almonds, the all-rounders** (page 20)
- **WAY 44: Honey, honey** (page 116)

Tip: As soon as you feel the first symptoms of a cold virus coming on, take black elderberry tincture in a glass of water twice or three times a day for a few days until symptoms subside. If you already have a full-blown cold, however, it's too late for this folk remedy!

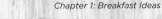

Blueberry-Orange Breakfast Dessert

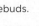

Try me out

A weekend 'special' to feast your eyes as well as your tastebuds.

Ingredients

400g live organic dairy
or soya yoghurt

Maple syrup or honey to taste

2 cups fresh blueberries

Peeled sections from 2 large oranges*

$1/4$ cup soaked or chopped nuts of choice

* To section an orange: peel the orange with a paring knife, thoroughly removing white pith, then slice between the membranes and lift individual segments out.

Serves 4

Method

1. Combine the yoghurt and maple syrup in a small bowl, stirring until blended.
2. Put $1/4$ cup blueberries into each of four tall glasses.
3. Spoon about 2 $1/2$ tablespoons of the yogurt mixture over the blueberries in each glass.
4. Add a few orange segments to each serving. Repeat layers with remaining blueberries, yogurt mixture, and oranges.
5. Sprinkle 1 tablespoon of chopped nuts over each serving and serve immediately.

WAY 5

Breakfast creations

As an alternative to commercial breakfast cereals high in added salt and sugar, create your own lavish brand of *muesli extraordinaire* with ingredients you have available at home.

Pre-soak a handful of porridge oats in filtered water (for 20 minutes or overnight), add some fresh seasonal fruit, pour milk or yoghurt over the top and decorate with seeds and nuts. For a deluxe version, sprinkle with coconut flakes, goji berries or raw chocolate nibs.

Porridge is another breakfast favourite: nourishing, cheap and so quick to make. A type of rice porridge called labazhou was considered a holy food in China during the Ming Dynasty and used in traditional Chinese medicine to support the spleen, stomach and blood. The main ingredients were boiled rice, millet, chestnuts, dried dates, nuts and brown sugar. So fond are the Chinese of their porridge, they have produced a canned porridge drink for their health conscious, highly active business market.

Even Germanic tribes in the 1st century AD were enjoying simple oat porridge. It is low-fat and a rich source of fibre, encouraging a steady release of energy rather than an instant 'high', followed by the inevitable 'slump'. If sensitive to oats, you can easily make a porridge using cereal grains or flakes made from rice, millet, buckwheat or quinoa. These are readily available in health stores. Using one of the cereals flakes as a base, put a handful into a saucepan and cover the flakes with two cups of boiling water (some cereals soak up more water than others).

Simmer gently for 10 minutes, stirring occasionally. Finally, add a dash of milk or milk substitute such as soya milk to make the porridge creamy. Cinnamon, nutmeg or vanilla enhance the taste and you can do without added sugar which can make you feel sleepy later on. Finally, pour the porridge mix over a bowl of chopped fruit and sprinkle with nuts and seeds.

During the working week, when time is short, a protein shake is a tasty, quick and nutrient-dense alternative. Use a blender to combine any of the following: fresh soft fruits such as banana, mango, papaya, berries (frozen are nice) or pineapple. Add a cup of yoghurt, kefir, silken tofu or tahini. Sweeten with a little honey or agave syrup if necessary, and use coconut, soya or rice milk to thin the consistency. For a thicker shake, simply add 1 tbsp of ground flaxseed.

If you prefer a cooked breakfast, scrambling or poaching an egg accompanied with cooked tomatoes and a slice of toasted rye bread is a useful way of combining quality protein, fibre and the potent antioxidant lycopene*. Or you may fancy some grilled or baked fish, such as haddock and mackerel with a fresh Greek salad. On the mornings, however, when you really get stuck for time or energy, consider just taking a spoon and digging into a humble avocado, one of nature's best wholefoods and a perfect breakfast dish to set you up for the day.

SEE ALSO

- **WAY 42: Cinnamon, add some spice into your life** (page 112)
- **WAY 47: Seeds: all good things come in small packages** (page 122)

Millet Melée

A scrumptious high-protein alternative to oat porridge.

Ingredients

$^1/_2$ cup millet grains
(not flakes)
2 $^1/_2$ cups water
2 ripe pears, peeled
and chopped
5 dried apricots chopped
1 pinch sea salt
$^1/_4$ tsp cinnamon
150ml milk or milk alternative
1 tbsp sunflower seeds
1–2 tsp butter

Serves 4

Method

1. Heat a dry pot to medium temperature. Add the millet and stir with a wooden spoon taking care not to burn the grains. After a few minutes the grains will give off a nutty aroma.

2. Add water, pears, apricots, cinnamon and salt. Bring to a boil. Turn down heat and simmer for approximately 25 minutes, stirring occasionally.

3. When the millet is soft, mix in the sunflower seeds, butter and milk and stir until creamy. Serve hot or cold.

Try me out

Tip: To make a quick and easy fruit salad, combine a can of peaches or pineapple sweetened with apple or grape juice, add a variety of chopped fruit of your choice and a little fresh orange, tangerine or apple juice. Jazz it up with some pecan nuts and coconut flakes.

WAY 6

Bring on the buckwheat

Contrary to its name, buckwheat is not a wheat and entirely different to other grains. It is really a seed and closely related to rhubarb.

For those who need to avoid wheat or gluten, buckwheat is a useful alternative, but it should also be valued for its outstanding nutritional qualities.

Buckwheat has a nutty, earthy flavour and can be eaten in a variety of different ways. The seed can be ground and milled into flour and made into pancakes, crumpets or bread. In Japan, buckwheat is called soba, and soba noodles are served in soups or dipped into sauces. The Russians like to crush buckwheat kernels into small pieces called groats and toast them. The resulting 'kasha' is used for breakfast cereals or side dishes. Russian soldiers are fed buckwheat for strength and stamina, and in Germany it is a popular ingredient in porridge, soups and puddings. First grown in China, it was cultivated in many parts of the world and introduced to Europe in the 12th century by returning crusaders. Sadly, buckwheat was rejected in the 19th century in favour of wheat, although it is a hardy species and able to thrive in poor conditions.

Now this versatile plant is becoming increasingly popular. High in digestible protein, it contains all the eight essential amino acids the body cannot make. At the same time, it is high enough in complex carbohydrates and dietary fibre to satisfy appetites and fuel energy. It is an ideal low GI food and valuable for all those with an interest in maintaining a healthy weight and balanced blood sugar levels. Buckwheat is also a good source of B vitamins, zinc, copper, manganese, selenium and a number of interesting antioxidant compounds such as rutin, quercetin* and hyperin*. Diets rich in such antioxidants are associated with a lower incidence of age-related degenerative diseases.

The bioflavonoid rutin* is of particular interest, as it is rarely found in the edible part of plants, except in buckwheat and grapes. Rutin is used by plants as protection against ultraviolet radiation and pests. In the human body, rutin appears to have antioxidant, anti-inflammatory and anti-carcinogenic effects. It is thought to strengthen the walls of tiny blood vessels called capillaries and help the blood to circulate more effectively (16). Rutin is particularly useful for those suffering from high blood pressure. Often called the 'silent killer', high blood pressure usually causes no symptoms until complications develop. Dietary and lifestyle factors can do much to prevent or manage this condition.

Some people may develop a sensitivity to buckwheat products involving asthma, urticaria and digestive disorders. However, this appears to be more common in those with coeliac disease.

SEE ALSO
- **WAY 1: A taste of cherry** (page 18)
- **WAY 16: Butter is better** (page 54)

Buckwheat Pancakes

These gluten-free pancakes are wonderful with either a sweet or savoury topping.

Ingredients

2 cups buckwheat flour
1 egg (optional)
2 tbsp melted butter
600ml milk or milk alternative
Ghee or olive oil for cooking

Makes 6–8 pancakes

Method

1. Beat buckwheat flour with the egg, melted butter and milk to make the batter.
2. Leave to stand for an hour, then pour 2 tbsp of batter into an oiled pan and cook until golden, flipping or turning once.
3. Serve with apple sauce (preferably homemade!) or stewed cherries. For a savoury pancake, layer with fresh spinach leaves and grated cheese.

Try me out

Tip: Soak buckwheat kernels for a day, then rinse and sprout until they grow 'little tails'. Finally, dehydrate at 105°F (41°C) until dry and crunchy. You can also use the oven set to its lowest temperature leaving the oven door at least 2 inches open to improve air circulation. Dehydrated buckwheat keeps well in a glass jar and is tasty sprinkled over salads, or as a healthy breakfast cereal mixed with berries, chopped fruit and nuts.

WAY 7

Fire up your digestion with ginger

The Chinese philosopher Confucius was a great believer in the healing properties of ginger, and is said to have eaten it at every meal.

Confucius, born in China in 551 BC, was one of the most respected philosophers in Chinese history, shaping political and moral thinking for centuries to come. In the time of Confucius, success in life was measured in terms of an individual's inner development rather than his outer position or accomplishments. He suggested that rulers should take 'as much trouble to discover what was right, as lesser men take to discover what will pay'.

In China, ginger was traditionally used to treat digestive complaints such as stomach upset, diarrhoea and nausea. To this day, fresh, dried, candied or pickled ginger is a staple in the Chinese diet and in many herbal remedies.

Ginger is an odd-looking, knobbly root covered in pale brown skin with a strong, zingy taste, ideal for soups, sauces, salads, stir-fries and desserts. It is also a great natural preservative. Throughout the ages, ginger has been used to treat a great variety of conditions. Its antioxidant, antimicrobial* and anti-inflammatory effects are attributed to the interaction of a number of active and pungent compounds including gingerols* and shogaols* (17). Keep ginger handy to combat the flu and ease a sore throat. It is also considered a useful tonic for the entire digestive tract as it helps to stimulate digestive enzymes. Many cultures enjoy a tea brewed from fresh ginger after meals in order to ease digestion. The ancient Greeks wrapped a piece of ginger into a slice of bread after large meals. Over time, ginger was mixed into the bread, creating the first gingerbread. To make ginger tea, pour boiling water into a cup containing a little grated ginger. Let it steep for a few minutes and add honey and lemon juice to taste.

Ginger is particularly effective for motion sickness and may help to prevent nausea and vomiting – and you may find it incorporated into dishes and drinks (ginger ale) on cruise ships and airlines. If using beverages containing ginger for this purpose, ensure it contains actual ginger, not artificial flavourings. During pregnancy, short-term use (no longer than four days) of not more than 1g/day poses little risk, but long-term use for pregnant women is not recommended. People with gallstones, heart conditions, diabetes or those on blood-thinning medication should consume ginger under supervision of their health care provider.

The mild anti-inflammatory properties of ginger make it a popular treatment for arthritis in supplement form or as a massage oil, to provide relief from pain and swelling. The Chinese use it to stimulate the circulation and warm the body. It can induce sweating, thereby cleansing the whole system. Ginger has recently even been associated with improved working memory and cognitive function. Is it any wonder that wise Confucius lived to a ripe old age?

SEE ALSO
- **WAY 2: Almonds, the all-rounders** (page 20)
- **WAY42: Cinnamon, add some spice into your life** (page 112)
- **WAY44: Honey, honey** (page 116)

Gingerbread Muffins

A perfect high protein breakfast or snack food treat.

Ingredients

1 ¹/₂ cups ground almonds
1 ¹/₂ cups ground pecans
1 tsp baking powder
1 tsp cinnamon
1 tsp mixed spice
2 eggs
¹/₃ cup honey
1 x 5cm piece fresh ginger grated

Makes at least 12 muffins

Method

1. Grind almonds and pecans in a blender and pour the resulting meal into a large mixing bowl.
2. Add the baking powder, cinnamon and mixed spice and combine well.
3. Whizz up the eggs, olive oil, honey and grated ginger in the blender and pour over the nut 'flour'. Mix well with a wooden spoon until you get a stiff, sticky batter.
4. Grease a twelve-cup muffin tin and line with cupcake papers.
5. Drop a tablespoon at a time of the mixture into the muffin tin. Take care not to overfill.
6. Bake at 180°C (350°F) for 10–15 minutes. Let muffins cool for 10 minutes before turning out.

Tip: For convenience, cut and peel fresh ginger into 3cm pieces and freeze them in a food storage bag. To use, simply take out the required amount and grate from frozen.

Kefir, the fizzy yoghurt drink

The name kefir means 'feel good' in Turkish.

More than 3,500 fermented foods and beverages (milk, vegetable or fruit based) are produced worldwide, primarily in Asia, Africa and the Middle East. Fermentation is the ancient and economical art of preserving food through the action of lactic acid* bacteria, yeasts and their enzymes. Fermented foods are easy to digest, nutritious and they have long been associated with significant health benefits (18).

Kefir is a fermented milk drink, popular for centuries in Eastern Europe. Tribes in the Caucasus Mountains first described that the fresh milk they carried in their leather pouches occasionally fermented into a tasty, fizzy drink. Believed to promote good health and longevity, the refreshing beverage is rapidly gaining in popularity (19).

Produced from a grainy mother culture, the semi-hard gelatinous grains are strained out of the milk after fermentation, then used to start off another batch. Traditionally, kefir was made by adding the culture to camel's milk. Any milk alternative can be used, including milk from cows, goats, sheep, buffalo and also from milk substitutes such as soya, seeds or nuts. Some people even make coconut water kefir. It is a refreshing drink on its own or can be used as a nutritious base for smoothies, dips and dressings.

Kefir contains probiotics*, so-called 'friendly' bacteria, which are responsible for keeping our intestines healthy and disease-resistant. It is increasingly evident that a healthy intestinal ecosystem protects against bacterial and fungal infections, allergies, atopic conditions, digestive disorders and many other diseases. Kefir's microorganisms reduce inflammatory responses in the gut which may explain some of its beneficial effects (20). Whereas yoghurt contains transient beneficial bacteria, the 'friendly' bacteria in kefir appear to be more resilient at colonizing the human gut.

The refreshing effervescence of kefir is due to a small and harmless amount of carbon dioxide and alcohol from the fermentation process. It also contains vitamins, minerals* and proteins* which are already partially digested and therefore easy for the body to absorb. Many people with a sensitivity to dairy products find they can tolerate kefir, and it is an ideal food for infants, the elderly and those with digestive problems.

Kefir can be obtained in economical starter packs in powdered form. The starter is simply added to handwarm milk and left to ferment at room temperature for 18–24 hours. Alternatively, live kefir grains can be used as a starter culture and recovered for subsequent batches.

SEE ALSO
- **WAY 3: Apples are as good they say, better in fact** (page 22)
- **WAY 16: Butter is better** (page 54)

Kefir Pancakes

Kefir can be used as an alternative to sour cream
or buttermilk to make moist, fluffy, delicious pancakes.

Ingredients

2 cups kefir
2 cups plain flour (or gluten-free flour)
1 tsp baking soda
$^1/_2$ cup milk or milk alternative
1 tsp vanilla extract
2 eggs, lightly beaten
Ghee or olive oil for cooking
Sliced apples or bananas

Makes approximately 10 pancakes

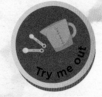

Method

1. In a large bowl, mix the dry ingredients together (flour and baking soda).
2. In a separate bowl, combine the kefir, milk, vanilla extract and eggs.
3. Add slowly to the dry mixture and mix gently until you get a lumpy batter.
4. Pre-heat a greased pan over medium heat and use a ladle to pour in the batter. Add sliced apples or bananas by pressing the thinly sliced fruit gently into the batter as the pancake is being cooked.
5. After 3–4 minutes, flip pancake over and continue cooking for a few minutes.
6. Serve with butter, fresh fruit or maple syrup.

Tip: Introduce kefir slowly, starting off with 4oz in the morning on an empty stomach and building up to a full 8oz glass daily.

9 Most definitely go to work on an egg

Eggs are one of the most affordable and best available sources of protein in a modern diet suffering from carbohydrate overload.

A medium-sized egg provides approximately 78 kcal and 6.5g of protein, delivering around 13% of an adult's daily protein requirement. Eggs are a complete protein source containing all amino acids essential for human health. They offer an excellent supply of vitamins D, B2 and B12, biotin*, iodine* and are a useful source of vitamin A, folic acid*, choline*, phosphorus* and selenium* (21).

The yolk in eggs contains large amounts of the carotenoids lutein* and zeaxanthin* which may reduce the risk of age-related macular degeneration. Eggs are also a good source of choline, a key nutrient for foetal development and useful 'brain food' as it aids memory and concentration, giving credence to the saying that one should, as the 1970's egg-promotion advertisement advised, 'go to work on an egg'. Over the last few decades, public confidence in eggs has been undermined by the worry over salmonella infections. Since the introduction of the Lion Quality Code of Practice in 1998, however, cases of salmonella in England and Wales have more than halved. Under the British Lion scheme, egg-producing hens must be vaccinated against salmonella – their eggs are always stamped with a red lion and a best-before date.

In order to decrease the risk even further, the Department of Health advises pregnant women not to eat raw or lightly cooked eggs. Discard cracked or dirty eggs, keep them refrigerated and eat them promptly after cooking. Always wash hands and cooking utensils after contact with raw eggs. Eggs can be given to babies over six months if thoroughly cooked. Some people are allergic to raw eggs, but may tolerate cooked eggs. Egg allergies are more common in children although many grow out of it.

In recent years, there has been a revision of dietary guidelines as studies have consistently demonstrated that eggs do not provide a risk for coronary heart disease when eaten as part of a healthy diet low in processed meats, saturated and trans fats and salt. Although eggs are a rich source of cholesterol, there is no recommended limit on how many eggs we can eat. The cholesterol from eggs has less effect on the amount of cholesterol in our blood than the amount of saturated fat*. Even those with high cholesterol do not appear to have a higher risk of heart disease or stroke if they regularly eat eggs. It should, however, be noted that people with familial hypercholesterolaemia, an inherited condition, have an increased sensitivity to dietary cholesterol and should restrict their egg consumption to two to three eggs per week.

SEE ALSO
- **WAY 22: Garlic is 'as good as ten mothers'** (page 66)

Tip: The best eggs come from healthy, well-nourished chickens. Look out for eggs from hens fed on flaxseed or fish-oil enriched feed, as they produce eggs with a higher omega-3 content, offering significant benefits to a heart-healthy diet.

Spanish Tortilla

Tortilla is a wonderful addition to picnics or lunchboxes.

Ingredients

6 eggs

1 1/2 pounds potatoes, peeled
and thinly sliced

2 tbsp olive oil

1 large onion, thinly sliced

Sea salt and freshly milled black pepper

2 cloves garlic, minced

2/3 cup milk or milk alternative

2 cloves garlic, minced

3 spring onions, chopped

1 cup grated cheddar cheese
(omit cheese if dairy intolerant)

Serves 2-3

Method

1. Preheat the oven to 180°C (350°F). In a large saucepan, simmer potato slices in water until just tender. Drain and reserve.

2. Heat the olive oil in a large non-stick saucepan and add the onion and garlic. Season to taste with sea salt and black pepper, and gently cook until soft, about five minutes. Remove the pan from heat.

3. In a large bowl, beat the eggs well, then stir in the milk, spring onions and cheese and combine until incorporated. Adjust the seasonings with salt and black pepper.

4. Add the onions and potatoes to the bowl and stir gently. Pour the entire mixture into an ovenproof casserole dish and bake until the eggs set, about 30 minutes. Serve warm or cold with a big green leafy salad.

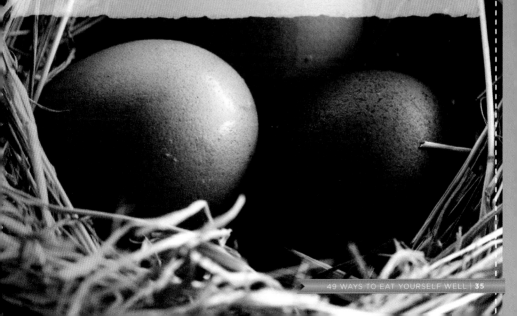

WAY 10 Oat cuisine

A slow-release complex carbohydrate is a power-packed breakfast that provides energy for the rest of the day – no wonder human beings have been eating oats for millennia!

It is surprising how many people skip breakfast, the most important meal of the day, and expect to keep going all morning without any fuel. By mid-morning, blood sugar levels may fall, causing faintness, irritability, lack of concentration and a craving for sugary, high-calorie convenience foods. This sets the pattern for the rest of the day – a trend towards eating unhealthy snacks or beverages containing substances which make us increasingly more tired.

Choose a balanced meal containing complex carbohydrates for energy plus some protein and essential fats. Even if you do not feel hungry first thing in the morning, it is important to replenish your food stores after an overnight fast, so keep it light and tasty. Oats offer unique nutritional properties and have been popular for millennia. Remnants of porridge have been found in the stomachs of 5,000-year-old bodies preserved in peat bogs in northern Europe. And for good reason – oats contain more protein and more unsaturated fats than most other cereal grains as well as high levels of beta-glucan*, a soluble fibre from the cell walls of the oat endosperm.

The US Food and Drug Administration have approved the health claim regarding the association between beta-glucan and a reduced risk of coronary heart disease. The proposed mechanism is that beta-glucan lowers the 'bad' LDL* and total cholesterol without affecting 'the good' HDL* cholesterol levels by binding to cholesterol-rich bile acids in the gut and promoting their excretion, rather than reabsorption into the body.

The soluble fibre from oats also improves glycaemic control* by delaying gastric emptying time and slowing down the absorption of glucose into the blood. Oats are therefore particularly useful for those wishing to control blood sugar levels and, due to their satiating properties, for those trying to maintain a healthy weight.

In addition, oats contain a number of unique anti-oxidant plant compounds called avenanthramides*. Researchers suggest these may provide valuable protection against a number of inflammatory conditions, including coronary heart disease, colon cancer and skin irritation (22).

Clinical evidence supports the view that some oat brands can be included in a gluten-free diet. Although the majority of oats may be contaminated with residues from gluten-containing cereals (wheat, barley, rye), gluten-free oat brands are now widely available. Create your own lavish brand of muesli with ingredients you have available at home: pre-soak some porridge oats in filtered water (overnight or even just for 20 minutes), add chopped fresh fruit (apples, pears, strawberries, peaches, berries), pour milk or yoghurt over the top and decorate with seeds and nuts. Fit for a king, yet affordable, healthy and easy on your digestion.

SEE ALSO

- **WAY 2: Almonds, the all-rounders** (page 20)
- **WAY 47: Seeds: all good things come in small packages** (page 122)

Perfect Porridge

Jazz up your porridge with fruit, seeds and nuts to make it even more nutritious and you will be tempted to eat it as a midnight feast as well as a comforting breakfast on colder days.

Ingredients

200ml rolled oats
400ml water
1 tsp butter
25g sunflower seeds
25g walnuts
$1/2$ apple, grated
Milk or milk substitute
Sea salt to taste

Serves 1

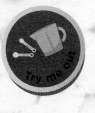

Method

1. Combine oats and water and bring to the boil. Add a pinch of sea salt.
2. Turn down the heat and let porridge simmer gently for 10 minutes.
3. Mix in a small knob of butter, sunflower seeds, walnuts and apple, and serve with cold milk.

Tip: Use an oatmeal bath to soothe, moisturise and cleanse the skin. Put two cups of rolled oats in a food processor (or coffee grinder) and grind into a powder. Add the oatmeal powder to a running bath of warm (not hot) water, stir well and soak in the bath for 15 minutes (take care as the bath will be slippery!).

WAY 11

Pineapple and its super-healing enzyme

Pineapples are versatile, juicy and delicious, are crammed with vitamins and minerals, and pack a powerful ingredient for healing.

Hurray for good old Christopher Columbus, who discovered and introduced us to such a variety of curious fruit and vegetables. In 1493 he stumbled upon a spiky-looking plant on the island of Guadeloupe. One of his crew described it as being 'in the shape of a pine cone, twice as big, which fruit is excellent and it can be cut with a knife, like a turnip and it seems to be wholesome' (23).

The explorers named it 'pina de Indes' and took it home to Spain. The exotic fruit was popular with sailors as its vitamin C content prevented scurvy. Later on, the English added the word 'apple'.

The pineapple has since become a worldwide favourite. Apart from vitamin C, the pineapple is full of fibre and the bone-building mineral manganese. Fresh pineapple juice is a traditional remedy for sore throats, and some boxing enthusiasts prefer to treat a black eye with a slice of fresh pineapple instead of raw steak.

Nutrition scientists show much interest in a compound called bromelain*, extracted from the stem of the pineapple plant. Bromelain is a proteolytic enzyme which means it is capable of digesting protein. When eaten directly after a meal, it aids the breakdown of proteins into amino acids. Fresh is best because the canning process deactivates the enzyme in the fruit. If you require assistance with your digestion but don't happen to be the fortunate owner of a pineapple plantation in the tropics, you can buy concentrated extracts of bromelain in tablet form from health food stores. The juice squeezed from a fresh pineapple also contains anti-inflammatory bromelain enzymes – although the juice is not as potent as bromelain–containing supplements.

Bromelain can also be used as a powerful natural anti-inflammatory agent without side-effects, and is popular for treating arthritic conditions. Bromelain also supports wound healing and is used effectively in treating sports-related injuries such as muscle tenderness, sprains and strains. It has a remarkable ability to reduce swelling and pain and increase joint mobility. If used for anti-inflammatory, rather than digestive purposes, it needs to be taken on an empty stomach between mealtimes. Please note that bromelain supplements are not suitable for those suffering from gastritis or ulcerative conditions of the stomach or colon.

Bromelain is less well known for its ability to improve respiratory ailments such as catarrh and bronchitis by reducing the viscosity of bronchial secretions. It has long been used in the treatment of sinusitis as an anti-inflammatory and mucolytic agent as it appears to thin nasal secretions and reduce inflammation of the nasal passages (24).

SEE ALSO

- **WAY 28: Nuts about coconuts** (page 78)
- **WAY 49: Versatile bananas for high energy** (page 126)

Pinemangonana Smoothie

A breakfast smoothie is high quality fuel-on-the-go.

Ingredients

1 cup pineapple
1 cup mango
1 banana frozen in chunks
$^1/_2$ cup coconut milk
$^1/_2$ cup water

Serves 2

Method

1. Pour coconut milk and water into a blender, then add the fruit and blend until smooth.
2. Add more liquid to reduce the thickness, ice to chill it, or use more fruit to thicken pineapple smoothie. Drink immediately.

Tip: To prepare a whole pineapple simply cut off the top, slice it in half lengthwise and then again. Remove the core, peel off the rind and cut into chunks for a fresh fruit salad. If you have any leftovers, spear them with a toothpick, freeze until solid and use as a treat for children.

WAY 12 Time for tea

The benefits of drinking tea were discovered around 4,000 years ago in ancient China.

Legend has it that Emperor Shen Nung was resting under a wild tea tree when a few tea leaves fell into his cup of boiling water, imbuing it with a delightful scent and flavour. The art of tea drinking also caught on in Japan, where green tea is considered an essential part of everyday life.

All varieties of black and green teas come from the plant Camellia sinensis. The difference between black and green tea is simply that black tea is produced from fermented leaves, whereas green tea retains its colour from unfermented leaves. Green tea contains a very high concentration of powerful anti-oxidants called polyphenols*. It has been extensively studied and reportedly lowers cholesterol, improves blood sugar control, boosts metabolism and burns fat. The predominant amino acid in green tea leaves, L-theanine*, when consumed regularly, helps to promote a state of relaxation and mental alertness. There is continuing interest in the potential health benefits of green tea for serious conditions including dementia, cancer, heart disease and inflammatory bowel disease.

Tea arrived in Britain just after the Middle Ages, and by the mid-18th century had become its most popular beverage – replacing ale for breakfast and gin at other times. However, a cup of tea infused for five minutes contains around 40mg of caffeine (half the amount found in a cup of coffee). Although caffeine does offer some health benefits, it is a mildly addictive stimulant which acts on the central nervous system affecting heart, muscles and digestive juices. This can promote restlessness or anxiety in some people and stress the adrenal glands. Another downside is that drinking tea with a meal reduces the absorption of iron* and zinc by up to 50%. This might pose a risk if already low in these minerals.

Rooibos (Redbush) tea is an excellent caffeine-free alternative and has a pleasantly aromatic, nutty flavour. The rooibos plant can only be cultivated naturally on the arid slopes of the Cedarberg mountain range in South Africa. It is particularly rich in flavonoids and minerals, and advocates claim it has anti-carcinogenic, anti-inflammatory and antiviral properties.

Herbal teas were possibly the first medicines ever invented and are still popular because they are effective and easy to use. Chamomile is one of my favourites. When Culpeper's famous 'Complete Herbal' was published in 1653, he stated that 'A decoction made of camomile taketh away all pains and stiches in the side... the bathing with a decoction of camomile taketh away weariness' (25).

Traditionally, chamomile tea has been used to relieve indigestion and can be used to stimulate the appetite when taken before mealtimes, especially in the aged. Diluted, it is said to ease wind and colic in infants. Chamomile also acts as a gentle sedative to soothe frazzled nerves and, at bedtime, may help those suffering with insomnia.

SEE ALSO

- **WAY 4: Berry healthy for you** (page 24)
- **WAY 8: Kefir, the fizzy yoghurt drink** (page 32)
- **WAY 42: Cinnamon, add some spice into your life** (page 112)
- **WAY 48: The wonderful world of flax** (page 124)

Green Tea Smoothie

A great way to incorporate your herbal teas!

Ingredients

1 cup freshly brewed green tea, cooled
$^1/_2$ cup frozen blueberries, blackberries
or raspberries
1 tbsp ground flaxseed
1 sweet whole fruit (such as banana,
peach, pear, apple, pineapple, mango)
$^1/_2$ cup live yoghurt or kefir*
$^1/_2$ tsp cinnamon

Serves 2

Method

Combine all ingredients and blend until smooth and creamy.

Try me out

Tip: Chamomile tea, when brewed strongly, can be used as a compress for treating skin conditions and to relieve itching. Reduce under-eye puffiness by soaking two chamomile tea bags in cool water and placing them over each eye.

RECIPE VARIATIONS
AND SUBSTITUTIONS

RECIPE VARIATIONS
AND SUBSTITUTIONS

RECIPE VARIATIONS
AND SUBSTITUTIONS

RECIPE VARIATIONS
AND SUBSTITUTIONS

1 2 3 4 5 6 7 8
9 10 11 12 **13 14**
15 16 17 18 19
20 21 22 23 24
25 26 27 28 29
30 31 32 33 34
35 36 37 38 39
40 41 42 43 44
45 46 47 48 49

Chapter 2

SALADS AND MAIN MEALS

From creamy soups to vibrant salads and tender roasted vegetables, here are ways to help you feel energized throughout the day. Whether planning a light packed lunch or a satisfying dinner, the emphasis is on protein-rich, high-fibre and nutrient-dense foods to stabilise blood sugar levels and boost your intake of anti-inflammatory plant compounds and healthy oils. Economical and simple to prepare, the recipe ideas have a special focus on improving digestive and immune health. Utilise fresh herbs as they are packed with nutrients and add a wonderful Mediterranean flavour to fish, meat and vegetable dishes.

WAY 13
Amaranth, the golden grain

When the Spanish plundered the Aztec and Inca civilisations in the 1500s, they also destroyed the natives' primary source of nutrition – amaranth.

Amaranth was believed to have magical medicinal properties and was incorporated into pagan Indian rituals including human sacrifice. The Spanish conquistadors were so appalled by this practice, they gave orders for all amaranth crops to be burned down and re-cultivation was forbidden. The highly nutritious plant might have become extinct if it had not survived in a few remote areas of the Andes and Mexico. Research in the 1950s identified its superior nutritional value, and amaranth was finally recognized as having major crop potential.

With ongoing famine worldwide, the race is on to find protein-rich grains. These need to be adaptable and easy to grow as well as resistant to heat, drought and disease. Amaranth not only fulfils all these criteria, but contains the highest protein values of any grain and is particularly rich in two essential amino acids, lysine and methionine.

Lysine is required for the production of collagen* and therefore the strength of tendons, ligaments, skin and other tissues. Methionine, one of the essential sulphur amino acids, contributes to the formation and the removal of important compounds in the body. Both amino acids are less commonly found in other grains.

Amaranth is also high in fibre and contains essential fatty acids, calcium, iron, potassium and vitamins A, C and E. The cooked grain is highly digestible and therefore valuable to infants and those recuperating from illness. It is ideal for gluten-free diets and vegetarians looking for a high quality protein source.

With such respectable nutritional credentials, it is surprising amaranth is not more commonly known and utilised. Amaranth has a sticky texture and care is needed not to use too much water or overcook. It has a pleasant, nutty taste and can be added to casseroles, soups, stews and stir-fries or cold-grain salads with chopped vegetables and toasted nuts. The small grains can be puffed like corn for cereals, flaked like oats for snacks, or finely ground to produce a gluten-free flour.

Research from New Zealand (42) has found that by replacing traditional flour such as wheat in breakfast cereals with amaranth, millet or buckwheat flours, it is possible to lower the glycaemic response. Low glycaemic foods can be used in addition to other strategies in the prevention of Type 2 diabetes, heart disease, obesity and cancer.

SEE ALSO
- **WAY 47: Seeds: all good things come in small packages** (page 122)
- **WAY 17: Cayenne pepper: some like it hot** (page 56)
- **WAY 31: Parsley, the potent free radical fighter** (page 84)

Amaranth Power Balls

Delicious served with stir-fries or brown rice with or without a tomato sauce, these power balls also work well with meat and fish dishes instead of potatoes. Can be eaten cold and added to your lunchbox salad.

Ingredients

$3/4$ cup amaranth grains
$1 1/2$ cups (400 ml) water
$1/2$ tsp vegetable bouillon
1 can (400g) cannellini beans mashed
(other bean varieties can also be used)
1 cup carrot steamed and finely chopped
(or use vegetable pulp from a juicer)
$1/2$ cup ground sunflower seeds
2 tbsp ground flax seeds
1 tbsp finely chopped onion
2 tsps parsley (fresh or dried)
or mixed herbs
2-3 tsps Tamari soy sauce
$1/2$ tsp dill
$1/4$ tsp each of sea salt and garlic pepper
3 pinches of cayenne pepper

Makes 16–20 power balls,
depending on size

Method

1. Add amaranth, water and vegetable bouillon to a saucepan and cook gently according to instructions on packet (around 30 minutes).
2. Once cooked, add the beans, carrot, onion, herbs, tamari, salt and peppers to the saucepan and mash well.
3. Combine the sunflower, pumpkin and flax seeds in a blender and grind to a flour. Add to the saucepan and mix thoroughly.
4. Shape into two-inch balls and place on a well-oiled baking tray. Bake for 20 minutes at 190°C (375°F).

Try me out

Tip: Place a layer of amaranth seeds into a preheated pan. Shake the pan gently until the seeds pop. Eat the puffed seeds as a nutritious snack, a cereal or as a crunchy topping for desserts.

14 Apple cider vinegar, an extraordinary nutritional drink

Who needs a cheap weightloss remedy that also doubles as a digestive aid? I guess many of us do. Here it is!

Vinegar is an ancient folk remedy that appears to have stood the test of time. The Babylonians used vinegar as a preservative and disinfectant, and in ancient Greece, Hippocrates prescribed it as a cure for various ailments. The Roman army supplied soldiers with 'posca', a thirst-quenching mixture made from vinegar and water, to provide them with energy on their arduous marches. In Japan, vinegar is still a popular tonic to reduce fatigue and improve circulation.

It has long been suggested but not yet conclusively proven that vinegar aids in weight control. Researchers in Sweden discovered one possible reason: they found that vinegar reduces the body's blood glucose and insulin response to carbohydrates, inducing a feeling of 'fullness'. Taking between two and three tablespoons of vinegar with a meal was associated with significantly lower blood sugar and insulin responses than having a meal without vinegar (26). An increased feeling of satiety is an added bonus for all those wanting to lose weight.

Apple cider vinegar is made from the fermentation of the juices of apples. In the first stage of fermentation, the sugars are turned into alcohol. In the second stage,

as the alcohol ferments further, vinegar is produced. When buying vinegar, always look for unfiltered organic apple cider vinegar. It is best to avoid low quality, highly refined vinegars labelled 'distilled' or those with added clarifiers, enzymes and preservatives.

Traditionally, apple cider vinegar is well established as a digestive aid that helps to acidify the stomach and break down proteins more efficiently. A lack of stomach acid is a common complaint and can lead to indigestion and sluggish digestion. Taking one tablespoon of the vinegar in half a glass of water after main meals may provide relief. Alternatively, eating a fresh, raw salad with a vinegary dressing before your meal may also be helpful. Diluted vinegar, however, should not be consumed by those suffering from excess stomach acidity, stomach ulcers or any other digestive disorders.

According to folklore, there may be countless health benefits to be gained from regularly consuming apple cider vinegar. Traditionally known as a detoxifier that helps to normalise the body's acid/alkaline balance, it is believed to be good for the circulation, provide relief from arthritic conditions and cleanse the digestive tract. It contains acetic acid and other acids, vitamins, minerals and amino acids. You can gargle with it or apply vinegar topically to disinfect cuts, wounds, insect bites and jellyfish stings.

SEE ALSO
- **WAY 29: Olives and the Mediterranean diet** (page 80)

Apple Cider Vinegar Dressing

You can give your dressing an extra 'tang' by
adding a tablespoon of balsamic vinegar.

Ingredients

1 cup of olive oil
1/2 cup of organic apple cider vinegar
1 tbsp Dijon or wholegrain mustard
2-3 cloves of garlic, finely minced
1/2 teaspoon each of fresh or
dried thyme and basil
A generous pinch
of sea salt and black pepper
1/2 tsp of honey

Method

1. Combine all ingredients except olive
   oil in a screw top jar and stir.
2. Add the olive oil, cover tightly
   with the lid and shake well.
3. Serve over your favourite raw salad.
   If stored, tightly covered, in the
   fridge, this dressing will keep for
   extended periods.

Try me out

Tip: Apple cider vinegar is highly acidic and should always be diluted with water or juice. Be aware that vinegar can erode your tooth enamel if you consume it on a daily basis, so always rinse your mouth with water after consuming it!

WAY 15

Broccoli and the astonishing crucifers

In Ancient Roman times, broccoli was developed from wild cabbage and its name is derived from the Latin 'bracchium' which means 'branch'.

With an ageing population, the incidence of cancer increases, and as this disease takes many years to develop, it is sensible to think about prevention. We can reduce known risk factors as much as possible, for instance being very overweight and avoiding exposure to cigarettes, alcohol, radiation and industrial carcinogens. However, it is not always possible to know the identity of cancer-causing agents, so a useful strategy is to find dietary sources of compounds that increase our cancer protection, well before any clinical symptoms become apparent.

This super veggie provides a complex range of tastes and textures and its colour can range from dark green to purple depending upon the variety. Broccoli is high in dietary fibre and contains beta carotene, folate, iron, calcium and potassium and excellent levels of vitamin C. The darker the florets, the higher the amounts of vitamin C and beta carotene. Broccoli is also a rich source of flavonoids such as kaempferol which appear to have a wide range of benefits, including anti-oxidant, anti-inflammatory and anti-allergic effects.

Cruciferous vegetables such as broccoli, brussels sprouts, cabbage, turnips, bok choi, kale, cauliflower, watercress and rocket all contain sulphur-containing compounds called glucosinolates. There is evidence to suggest that a high intake of these valuable phytochemicals* reduces the risk of developing cancer, in particular lung and colorectal cancer. Much more research, however, is required and the influence of genetic factors also needs to be taken into account (27).

Once eaten, the glucosinolates from crucifers are converted in the mouth and digestive tract to biologically active compounds that not only improve our ability to detoxify carcinogens, but may also activate tumour suppressor genes. Of all the cruciferous vegetables, broccoli appears to have the highest levels of glucosinolates. One of the most potent of these is the organosulphur compound sulforaphane. When chewing broccoli (or other crucifers), plant enzymes transform the largely inactive glucosinolates into the active sulforaphane. Our intestinal bacteria in the lower gut also help to increase sulphoraphane absorption.

Researchers have discovered that different commercial varieties of broccoli vary significantly in the amount of glucosinolates they contain. They also discovered that the fresher the vegetable, the more phytochemicals present. To make use of the natural anti-cancer agents found in crucifers, eat a generous portion of broccoli at least three times a week and re-use the cooking water, as the active compounds are water-soluble. Raw broccoli contains considerably more glucosinolates than cooked broccoli, so if you are going to cook it, lightly steamed is best.

SEE ALSO
- **WAY 22: Garlic is 'as good as ten mothers'** (page 66)
- **WAY 18: Celery, a dose of Hippocrates's medicine** (page 58)

Broccoli and Cauliflower Chowder

A nourishing and comforting soup, simple to make and eat.

Ingredients

1 tbsp butter
1 tbsp extra-virgin olive oil
1 medium onion, chopped
1 stalk celery, chopped
1 large potato chopped
2 cloves garlic, minced
8 cups chopped broccoli and cauliflower (stems and florets)
400g can cannellini beans (rinsed)
6 cups water
1 tsp vegetable bouillon
Freshly ground pepper to taste

Serves 4-6

Method

1. Heat butter and oil in a large saucepan over medium heat until the butter has melted. Add onion, garlic, celery and potato and cook, stirring occasionally, for about five minutes.
2. Stir in broccoli, cauliflower and beans. Then add the water and bouillon and simmer gently for about 10 minutes or until the vegetables are tender.
3. Puree the soup in batches in a blender until smooth and creamy. Use caution when pureeing hot liquids. Season to taste and serve.

Tip: The health value of broccoli decreases significantly if cooked until soft and mushy. Lightly stir-fry for two or three minutes, or steam until still a little crunchy. Don't throw away the broccoli stalks – juice them or add to soups and casseroles.

WAY 16

Butter is better

It is difficult to establish when butter was first produced, although it was mentioned in the Old Testament, and in records as early as 2,000 BC.

Over the centuries, butter has been revered for its nutritional, medical and even cosmetic qualities. Ancient Asiatic tribes enjoyed its taste and smeared it on their skin to protect them from the cold. The Greeks and Romans rubbed butter into their hair to make it shiny, and it has long been used to treat skin infections, burns and as a soothing remedy for sore throats.

Butter is a milk fat provided from cows, sheep, goats, camels or water buffalo. Methods of butter production have been many and varied, but the most innovative, surely, was to place the cream from milk in a bag behind the saddle of a horse and ride until the butter-making process was complete. The churning of cream must have been a tedious and wearisome process typically accomplished by hand and a wooden churn. Now of course the production of butter is a carefully controlled operation; the first butter factories were built in the 19th century.

The nutritional qualities of butter justify its popularity, particularly if sourced from grass fed, pastured and contented cows – unlike highly processed vegetable oils or butter substitutes which may contain trans fats, synthetic vitamins, emulsifiers, artificial flavours, solvents or preservatives.

In addition to the fat-soluble vitamins A, E and K, butter contains vitamin D which is essential for the absorption of calcium and necessary for the development of healthy bones and teeth. Butter is one of the few foods that supplies iodine in a highly absorbable form, as well as selenium. Both of these minerals are critical for thyroid function.

Butter also provides useful amounts of short- and medium-chain fatty acids which are easy to digest and absorb for energy. Butyric acid, a short-chain fatty acid found in butter is required as the primary energy source for the cells of our intestinal membranes, and helps to maintain the integrity of the gastrointestinal wall. There is some evidence that high levels of butyric acid may reduce chronic inflammation of the colon.

Medium-chain fatty acids provide an immediate source of energy and are therefore popular with endurance athletes, such as long distance swimmers. Conjugated linoleic acid (CLA) is another naturally-occurring fatty acid that is particularly high in butter from livestock allowed to forage on grass. Claims that CLA helps to improve immune function and reduce body weight still need to be confirmed in human trials. All dairy products contain the milk sugar lactose, although butter only contains traces of lactose and may not cause problems for lactose-intolerant individuals. However, those with an allergy to milk need to avoid it.

Clarified Butter Recipe

Clarified butter (also called ghee) is an excellent choice for frying and sautéing as its chemical structure is more stable than butter or vegetable oil.

To make clarified butter, put a lump of butter in a stainless steel or glass dish and place in the oven at a low temperature until melted. Remove the whitish residue (the milk solids) by skimming it off or pouring through a strainer lined with cheese-cloth.

Store the clear 'golden' butter oil in a glass jar and use for cooking.
It keeps for extended periods without going rancid if kept in the fridge.

Tip: Mix $1/2$ cup softened butter with 2 tbsp cold-pressed flaxseed oil and 2 tbsp extra virgin olive oil for easier spreading.

WAY 17

Cayenne pepper – some like it hot!

Cayenne pepper is a popular herb known for adding extra 'zing' to hot and spicy dishes, but few realise its great health promoting potential.

The spice is not related to black pepper but is made from a variety of red hot chilli peppers native to Central and South America. Paprika is a milder version of cayenne pepper.

Herbalists consider cayenne to be one of the safest and most potent stimulants with a wide variety of applications wherever there are symptoms of coldness or stagnation. It has been used for centuries as a remedy for weak digestion, encouraging the output of gastric juices and thereby improving the function of the entire digestive system. Other traditional uses include boosting blood circulation, warding off colds and clearing headaches and sinus problems.

Applied topically, cayenne pepper can help to relieve muscle and arthritic pain. The active ingredient, capsaicin, causes a warm glow on initial application and may linger for about 30 minutes before it subsides. When using cayenne in form of capsaicin ointment, ensure you don't let it come into contact with irritated skin or open wounds and keep it away from your eyes and nose. If this does happen, the burning sensation may be intense, but is harmless and transient and best washed away with water and vinegar. If the fiery sensation occurs in the mouth, sip a little milk.

Other important ingredients include vitamins A and C, and flavonoids and carotenoids, pigments which have anti-oxidant properties and provide plants with their beautiful colours.

Adding cayenne to food may help to suppress appetite and burn calories. A study has found that half a teaspoon of cayenne pepper mixed in with a meal burns an extra 10 calories compared to eating the same meal without it. It was also found that some people, particularly those who were not regular consumers of cayenne, experienced a reduction in appetite (28). The novice cayenne pepper user, however, would be wise to start off with small amounts such as a tip of a teaspoon, as the intensity of symptoms from larger doses might indeed put you off your dinner.

Please note that if you are currently being treated with prescribed medication, you should not use cayenne pepper in large amounts without first talking to your doctor or nutritionist.

SEE ALSO
- **WAY 16: Butter is better** (page 54)
- **WAY 22: Garlic is 'as good as ten mothers'** (page 66)

Tip: For sore throats and colds: at the onset of symptoms, add $1/4$ teaspoon of cayenne pepper to a glass of warm water with the juice of a lemon and a teaspoon of honey. Stir thoroughly, use as a gargle and drink slowly. Cayenne pepper helps to promote detoxification by causing the skin to sweat, the eyes to water and nose to run.

Red Cayenne Pepper Soup

A rich and warming winter soup with a vibrant colour.
Go easy on the cayenne if unused to it.

Ingredients

4 large red bell peppers
1 onion, chopped
2 potatoes, peeled and diced
2 cloves garlic, chopped
600ml vegetable or chicken stock
1 tbsp butter
Cayenne pepper, black pepper and
sea salt

Serves 2–3

Method

1. Wash and cut the red bell peppers
   in half and remove the seeds.
2. Baste in olive oil and roast in a
   pre-heated oven at 200°C (400°F)
   for about 30 minutes.
3. Remove peppers from the oven and let
   them cool down. Remove any blackened
   skin with a sharp knife.
4. Heat the butter in a large soup pot over
   medium-high heat, add the chopped
   onions, potatoes, garlic and roasted
   peppers. Stir well and cook gently
   for 5–10 minutes.
5. Add the stock, stir well and bring to
   a simmer. Cook over a medium heat
   until potatoes are soft, then purée the
   soup in a blender or food processor
   until very smooth.
6. Season and add cayenne pepper
   according to taste.

WAY 18

Celery, a dose of Hippocrates's medicine

The physician Hippocrates, born in 460 BC on the Greek Island of Cos, stated 'let food be thy medicine and let thy medicine be food'.

He believed in the natural healing processes of diet, rest, fresh air and cleanliness – and that the body should be treated as a whole rather than a series of different parts. The 'Father of Medicine' developed an Oath of Medical Ethics taken by many doctors as they begin their medical practice. But these days, you are unlikely to be handed a stick of celery as you walk into any surgery, and more likely to be told 'let thy medicine be anti-depressants and high blood pressure tablets'.

So let us examine that stick of celery to see what it can do for us. Wild celery was first known as a medicinal herb rather than a vegetable. In Ancient Greece, it was revered as a holy plant and the green leaves fashioned into laurels to decorate winning athletes. Hippocrates used celery to treat anxiety and the essential oils in celery seeds do appear to have a calming effect on the central nervous system.

Hippocrates also used the seeds to increase the flow of urine. The diuretic properties of celery along with its anti-bacterial and anti-inflammatory compounds make it a useful and popular treatment for urinary tract infections. Celery is also recommended for gout sufferers as it aids in the removal of excess uric acid, a chemical that can trigger painful gout attacks. In addition, the insoluble fibre in celery stalks helps to prevent constipation by speeding up the passage of food and waste through the gut.

Celery contains significant amounts of potassium and organic sodium which regulate fluid balance. In China, where the health benefits of celery were first documented in the 5th century AD, clinical studies have demonstrated that celery seeds from the flowers of the plant may lower blood pressure.

Active compounds called phthalides relax arterial muscles, allowing them to dilate, thereby reducing blood pressure (29). It is worth buying organic to avoid pesticides and also noting that celery should not be eaten in large quantities by pregnant women, people with acute kidney inflammation or anyone on diuretics without first seeking medical approval.

Did you know that the celery plant is related to carrots, parsnips and parsley? Enjoy fresh celery by adding its leaves or sliced stalks to salads, soups, stews and stir-fries. The next time you juice carrots, add a celery stalk, particularly if suffering from a hangover. And here is a fine formula from the 1600s for any budding witches, 'Eat celery seeds so that you won't get dizzy when flying about on your broom'. Harry Potter would do well to take note.

> **Tip: Celery is a natural diuretic. Eating raw celery or juicing raw organic celery stalks regularly is beneficial for the cardiovascular system as it may help to lower blood pressure. For a really tasty snack, cut celery stalks into 3-inch (8 cm) lengths and fill the hollow with nut butter.**

Veggie Waldorf Salad

Waldorf Salad is a perfect winter or summer salad: sweet, crunchy and punchy. You can use raisins instead of grapes and pecans instead of walnuts. For vegetarians or those intolerant to eggs, the veggie mayo is as appetising as real mayonnaise.

Ingredients

$1/2$ cup chopped walnuts
$1/2$ cup chopped celery
$1/2$ cup red seedless grapes, sliced
1 chopped apple
3–4 tbsp veggie mayonnaise (see below)
Sea salt and black pepper to taste
Lettuce leaves (optional)

Method

In a medium-sized bowl, combine the celery, grapes, and walnuts. Add apple last to prevent it from browning. Mix in the veggie mayo, seasoning and serve immediately on a bed of fresh lettuce.

Serves 2

Veggie Mayonnaise

Ingredients

1 cup cashew (or macadamia) nuts
$1/2$ cup water
4 tbsp olive oil
3 tbsp lemon juice
Pinch of sea salt
1–2 tbsp of balsamic vinegar

Method

Blend all ingredients except the balsamic vinegar in a high speed blender until smooth. Add the balsamic vinegar and blend again until the 'mayonnaise' thickens.

Serves 2

WAY 19

Cherish the chickpea, a multi-talented bean

Chickpeas (or garbanzo beans) are practical, cheap, versatile and always useful to have in your store cupboard.

Sandy in colour, chickpeas have a pleasingly nutty flavour to complement salads, stir-fries and soups. Properly prepared, these legumes are highly nutritious and a staple food in many parts of the world.

In the Middle East where they originated, chickpeas are used to make hummus and falafel balls, while the flour of ground chickpeas, also known as gram flour, is popular in India for use in pancakes and pastry.

Frequent consumption of legumes is known to have a beneficial effect on health, with regular consumption reducing the risk of heart disease, cancer and Type 2 diabetes. The humble chickpea has, in animal studies, been found to lower cholesterol and improve blood sugar levels, and can be used as a functional food for diabetics and insulin-resistant individuals due to its high protein and fibre content (30). Research is also currently underway to develop chickpea-based milk powder and baby foods for infants that are unable to tolerate dairy or soya.

Chickpeas are a good source of folic acid and the minerals manganese, iron, copper, zinc and magnesium. Sprouting chickpeas is easy, tasty and substantially increases their content of available vitamins B and C. Chickpeas also contain phytoestrogens which may affect the body's own production of oestrogen, potentially lowering the risk of breast cancer, protecting against osteoporosis and reducing hot flushes in post-menopausal women.

Increased consumption of higher fibre foods is also associated with improved bowel health and stool consistency. Chickpeas are high in insoluble fibre which passes undigested through the digestive tract until it undergoes bacterial fermentation in the large intestine. The resulting products of fermentation are short-chain fatty acids (SCFAs), used by cells lining the intestine as a preferred source of energy. Butyric acid is one of the most potent SCFAs and thought to be a protective factor in colon cancer. Some people may experience increased flatulence after consuming chickpeas. Ensure therefore, that they are well-soaked and well-cooked (old chickpeas take longer to cook).

For convenience, use the canned version, although canned chickpeas contain higher levels of sodium than freshly cooked ones. To cook dried chickpeas, soak them in a large bowl of cold water overnight (12 hours), rinse well then put them into a large pot and cover with plenty of water. Bring to a boil, then cover and simmer for one to two hours, until the chickpeas are tender.

SEE ALSO
- **WAY 22: Garlic is 'as good as ten mothers'** (page 66)
- **WAY 25: Lemon Aid** (page 72)
- **WAY 29: Olives and the Mediterranean diet** (page 80)

Speedy Hummus

Beautifully creamy, with a hint of citrus and a lovely nutty taste.

Ingredients

400g can of chickpeas
4 tbsp lemon juice
3 cloves of garlic, finely minced
1 tsp cumin
Sea salt, freshly ground black pepper
100ml tahini
(sesame seed paste)
6 tbsp water
4 tbsp extra virgin olive oil
1 tsp paprika

Makes about 2 cups

Method

1. Drain the chickpeas and rinse well.
2. Combine the chickpeas, lemon juice, garlic, cumin, salt, pepper, tahini and water in a food processor or blender and process to a creamy consistency.
3. Add more lemon juice, garlic and seasoning to taste. Sprinkle with paprika and serve with pitta bread, falafel or crudités.

Try me out

Tip: Roasted chickpeas make a tasty savoury snack. Drain and rinse canned or freshly cooked chickpeas. Mix with some olive oil, tamari soy sauce and favourite seasonings. Spread chickpeas on a baking sheet and place in a preheated oven. Roast for 30 minutes at 200°C (400°F), shaking the pan regularly to allow them to brown evenly.

20

Chicken soup for the soul... and the nose

Meat broths and stocks are nutritious, comforting and easy to swallow and digest.

Good homemade stock can be made by boiling up the bones and cartilage from beef, lamb, chicken or fish with vegetables, herbs and spices. Nothing goes to waste as you can drink the broth or use it to enrich soups, stews, sauces and rice dishes. Meat stocks concentrate the flavours and nutrients from their ingredients, and consumed on a daily or regular basis, many people believe they offer protection from a variety of health complaints (31). When I was a child, my German-born mother would make nourishing chicken broths whenever we were ill, and I am sure they contributed to many a quick recovery!

There is an old wives' tale that traditional chicken soup is a useful cold remedy and natural decongestant, which may yet turn out to be true. In the 12th century, the Jewish physician Moses Maimonides prescribed chicken soup as a treatment for colds and asthma, declaring that chicken soup 'is recommended as an excellent food as well as medication' (32). Although there is only limited scientific evidence for this, a study in 2000 found chicken soup did indeed reduce upper respiratory symptoms (33).

The soup used in the study contained chicken, onions, sweet potatoes, parsnips, turnips, carrots, celery stems, parsley, salt and pepper. It appears that no single compound on its own is responsible for loosening congestion. The combination of all ingredients working together is likely to be the therapeutic factor.

Minerals from the bones, cartilage, marrow and vegetables are easy to absorb and chicken contains the amino acid cysteine which is released into the soup, aiding the breakdown of mucous in the respiratory tract.

Meat-based stocks, broths or bouillons are much more than just cold remedies. Records from 18th century Germany reveal that meat stocks were used for wasting diseases, dysentery and hyperacidity of the stomach. During the slow simmering process, the cartilage from joints and the marrow from bones are gradually incorporated into the broth. Cartilage contains collagen which has been used to treat digestive disorders for centuries and is also believed to improve skin, promote wound healing, and strengthen connective tissue and bones. Bone marrow is the soft substance found inside bones and contains protein, healthy fats, vitamins and minerals as well as important immune factors. It appears to have been much prized by our ancestors in the Stone Age (34). They did not waste food resources and went to great lengths to break open the bones of their prey and feast on the rich marrow.

Once chilled, meat stocks set as a soft jelly and can be kept in the fridge for up to a week, or frozen for up to six months. Commercially available soups, bouillons and stock cubes are best avoided as they are generally high in sodium and additives.

SEE ALSO
- **WAY 22: Garlic is 'as good as ten mothers'** (page 66)
- **WAY 31: Parsley, the potent free radical fighter** (page 84)
- **WAY 18: Celery, a dose of Hippocrates's medicine** (page 58)

Simple Chicken Broth

This is a soup to make in advance and have at your leisure, for pleasure!
Longer cooking provides a richer, more nutritious broth.

Ingredients

1 whole free-range chicken (1.5 kg)
3 litres of cold filtered water
(approximately)
2 tbsp vinegar
5-10 peppercorns
1 large onion,
coarsely chopped
2 carrots, peeled
and coarsely chopped
3 celery stalks,
coarsely chopped
Small bunch of parsley
2 tbsp garlic, chopped

Serves 8-10

Method

1. Place chicken in a pot with cold water, vinegar and all vegetables except the parsley and garlic.
2. Bring slowly to a boil, reduce heat, cover and simmer for an hour until meat is tender.
3. Carefully remove the whole chicken with a slotted spoon and take off the meat, reserving it for later or for use in sandwiches, rice or pasta dishes.
4. Place the bones back into the stock and simmer for at least a further hour, preferably 3-4 hours.
5. Strain the stock by pouring the soup through a sieve into a separate pot to remove bones, vegetables and peppercorns.
6. Add the parsley and garlic and simmer for a further 10 minutes. Keep the stock in the fridge or freezer and record the date and type of stock on the label.
7. To make a soup, add a variety of chopped vegetables to the stock and simmer for 15 minutes. Just before serving add some of the reserved and chopped chicken and heat through.

Try me out

Tip: Add vinegar, acidic wine or lemon juice to your stock pot at the beginning of cooking to draw minerals such as calcium, magnesium and potassium into the broth (add 2 tbsp per 2 lbs of bones). Beef and lamb bones contain more bone marrow than chicken and provide a tastier broth if roasted in the oven before cooking.

WAY 21 Fish for the brain

The Moken are one of the last surviving nomadic populations. Also known as 'sea-gypsies', they live around the coastal areas of Southeast Asia.

The Moken lead the traditional life of the hunter–gatherer, taking advantage of the incredible variety of marine life. Living on wooden boats, they sail from island to island using nets, traps and spears to catch fish, molluscs, sandworms, shells, sea snails and other sea creatures. During the monsoon time, they work on the seashore, repairing their boats and selling nutritious bounty from the sea.

Moken children are born in the water and wean themselves by swimming down to the seabed to forage for seafood. These children are excellent divers with a remarkable ability to see clearly underwater (35). According to Professor Michael Crawford (Imperial College, London), an eminent researcher into brain function and nutrition, this is mainly due to their diet, in particular the essential lipid DHA found in the marine food chain, and a genetic inheritance reinforced by the diet of their ancestors (36).

DHA is particularly important for brain structure during early brain development. Seafood also provides a useful source of protein, vitamins and many important trace elements. When the 2004 tsunami hit the region, the Moken predicted its arrival and were able to escape in time. Through the ages, the Moken have been exploited and pursued by 'civilised' society.

Only around 5,000 Moken survive today and are resisting attempts to be permanently housed and exhibited as tourist attractions.

In the UK, we have seen a huge increase in learning problems, anti-social behaviour, mood and neurological disorders. No attention is paid to the essential role of diet in the official assessment or management of such conditions. Nutritionists are concerned about people consuming the 'right' fats, because it has long been established that essential fatty acids, obtained from food, are vital for brain development. Omega-3 fats in fish provide key building blocks for the brain, nerve membranes and the retina of the eye and help to carry messages between nerve cells. They are also involved in helping to reduce the risk of heart disease and strokes, and relieving the inflammatory symptoms of auto-immune disorders.

Experts recommend that we should be eating two to four portions of fish per week, particularly oily fish such as salmon, sardines, pilchards, herring, trout or mackerel. Although some types of fish may carry contaminants, the benefits from consuming seafood are likely to outweigh any risks. Some people have higher dietary requirements for omega-3 than others, and it is therefore always important to rule out any omega-3 deficiencies with individuals suffering from behaviour, learning or mood disorders.

SEE ALSO
- **WAY 16: Butter is better** (page 54)
- **WAY 29: Olives and the Mediterranean diet** (page 80)

Baked Mackerel with Tomatoes

Wonderfully satisfying and tasty, this fish dish
supplies you with the ultimate brain food.

Ingredients

2 large mackerel, gutted and with heads
removed

12 red cherry tomatoes

3 tbsp balsamic vinegar

A little olive oil

Fresh basil leaves or two dried ones

2 tbsp butter

Sea salt and freshly ground black pepper

Serves 2

Method

1. Preheat the oven to 200°C (400°F). Rub the mackerel all over with a little olive oil, salt and black pepper. Place the mackerel in a baking dish.

2. Push the butter and basil into the inner cavity of each fish. Surround each fish with the tomatoes, splash with vinegar and drizzle with a little more oil. Cover.

3. Place on the middle shelf of the preheated oven for about 20 minutes, until the fish is tender. Serve with a traditional Greek salad.

Try me out

Tip: Try to ensure the fish comes from a sustainably managed source. The two major UK labels are the Marine Stewardship Council's (MSC) label and the Soil Association's organically farmed label. The new Aquaculture Stewardship Council (ASC) aims to be the world's leading certification and labelling programme for responsibly farmed seafood.

22

Garlic is 'as good as ten mothers'

Garlic, a member of the onion family and one of the best-known cure-alls, is, according to an old Indian proverb 'as good as ten mothers'.

But we tend to avoid it in large doses because of the unpleasant odour we emit after eating some. 'A nickel will get you on the subway, but garlic will get you a seat' is a saying from New York, perfectly capturing our dislike of its pervasive pong.

Our ancestors, however, knew a good remedy when they saw one. In ancient Egypt, garlic was so highly prized that pyramid workers went on strike when deprived of their daily garlic rations. The Romans dedicated the herb to Mars, the Roman god of war and ensured their armies were adequately supplied in order to improve strength and stamina. Garlic was believed effective in treating almost every common ailment, including scorpion stings, dog bites, respiratory problems, bladder infections and intestinal worms. On long marches, foot soldiers wedged fresh cloves between their toes to prevent fungal infections.

Although some may avoid garlic like the plague, people in the Middle Ages ate garlic to protect themselves against it. Modern scientific study has since found that garlic does indeed possess antibiotic, antifungal and antiviral properties and enhances the function of our immune cells. One imagines those eating it would have been so malodorous, nobody would have ventured close enough to spread the infection. Apparently, it worked a treat at warding off the odd vampire as well.

Garlic has long been known to support the cardiovascular system. Although unlikely to lower cholesterol and triglycerides as quickly as drugs, it may be safer for long-term use. Garlic also appears to inhibit platelet stickiness, reduce the risk of thrombosis and arterial plaque formation (37). Anyone on anti-coagulant medication or scheduled for surgery, however, should not use garlic in high doses because of its ability to thin the blood.

Both garlic and onions contain the amino acid cysteine which improves the bioavailability of iron and zinc from food grains such as rice and pulses (38). In addition, cysteine is capable of breaking down mucous, so garlic and onions can be used as natural decongestants during upper respiratory tract infections. An easy way of doing this is to peel and cut up an onion and leave it on a saucer by your bedside overnight.

The sulphur compound allicin is another key factor involved in garlic's healing properties and only becomes active once a clove is crushed, chewed or chopped. Once digested, allicin is eliminated via the lungs and skin and becomes responsible for garlic's pungent aroma.

One to two cloves of garlic a day is usually recommended and considered safe in adults. Be aware that eating raw garlic, particularly on an empty stomach, may cause heartburn, flatulence or digestive upset in some people.

SEE ALSO
- **WAY 31: Parsley, the potent free radical fighter** (page 84)

Roasted Garlic and Onion Soup

The ultimate soup for soupy weather: rich, smooth and comforting.

Ingredients

8 large garlic cloves with skins

3 large onions, sliced

2 tbsp olive oil

5 cups vegetable broth or bouillon

3 fresh thyme sprigs or $1/2$ tsp dried thyme

$3/4$ cup potato, peeled and diced

Fresh parsley, chopped

Serves 4

Method

1. Preheat oven to 160°C. Mix onions, garlic cloves and olive oil in a baking pan. Roast until garlic and onions are tender, about 30 minutes. Cool. Squeeze garlic out of skin and mash.

2. Put onions and garlic into a saucepan and add vegetable broth, diced potato, thyme and bring to a boil. Reduce heat and simmer for 15 minutes. Cool.

3. Puree soup in a blender and return to saucepan. Gently reheat and season to taste with sea salt and black pepper. Ladle soup into bowls, sprinkle with fresh parsley and serve.

Tip: To improve immune function and fend off colds, eat one clove of raw garlic/day. To reduce 'garlic breath', place the very finely chopped garlic onto a teaspoon and drop into the back of the mouth. Swallow the garlic with a little water and do not chew.

WAY 23

Healthy lunchbox ideas

It's a challenge not to succumb to convenience items in a time-driven society, such as crisps, fizzy drinks, chocolate bars and sweets so commonly found in lunchboxes or snack packs.

This type of refined diet is high in sugar, salt, unhealthy types of fat, artificial additives and low in fibre and vitamins, minerals and essential fatty acids – all necessary ingredients for health and vitality. Rather than the usual refined processed 'bread', make sandwiches with real, old-fashioned bread for lunch. Tasty artisan bread that is yeast-free, wheat-free, low in salt and made with organic wholegrain flour using slow fermentation processes can be found online and in selected stores. Some supermarkets are now carrying a range of artisan breads.

Protein fillers for wholemeal sandwiches or pitta bread pockets can include home-cooked beef, poultry or fish, hummus, tahini, falafel, cheese or eggs combined with a salad topping. Try out combinations of spinach and lettuce leaves, alfalfa sprouts, cucumber slices and grated carrot.

A good way to avoid the typical mid-afternoon slump is to enjoy a large mixed salad at lunchtime. Easy to digest, main-meal salads provide a rich source of vitamins, minerals, enzymes, essential fats, complex carbohydrates and fibre to keep energy levels stable. Vary the ingredients according to what you have at home and choose from different colours and textures, including fresh crunchy vegetables, seeds and grains. Leftover portions of rice, millet or quinoa from the night before can be made into

a tasty grain salad. Simply combine these in a large Tupperware container with a protein source (beans, tofu, nuts and seeds, a hard-boiled egg, fish or chicken) and add green leafy salad varieties with grated, chopped or sliced vegetables. Finally, drizzle a few tablespoons of home-made dressing over the top and remember to pack a fork!

Sprouted seeds and grains are full of goodness and add texture to salads. Easy to sprout seeds, grains and pulses include alfalfa, mung beans, chickpeas, lentils, sunflower, aduki and barley. Health food shops sell sprouter kits with full instructions. It is also simple and satisfying to grow your own sprouts with minimal equipment. Soak the seeds, pulses or grains for 12–24 hours, wash, drain, spread on a seed tray and stand on a sunny windowsill. Rinse twice daily and within a few days you can harvest the sprouts. Use the sprouted foods to sprinkle over your salads or add to cooked foods as a garnish.

As a sweet treat, fresh washed fruit is easy to carry and instant healthy fast food 'on the go'. Pears, peaches, apples, satsumas, grapes and cherries are all ideal. Home-made slices of almond bread, low-sugar oatmeal raisin biscuits, flapjacks, nuts or home-made popcorn are all healthy, energising lunchbox additions.

SEE ALSO

- **WAY 14: Apple cider vinegar, an extraordinary nutritional drink** (page 50)
- **WAY 34: Quinoa, an old food for the future** (page 90)
- **WAY 36: Spinach, iron and muscle strength** (page 94)
- **WAY 47: Seeds: the best things come in small packages** (page 122)

Rainbow Salad

This salad is all about taste and colour, so use your creativity.
Any combinations of salad leaves and vegetables can be used;
try to eat a rainbow of colours. Experiment and each salad will be different.

Ingredients

1 hard boiled egg (sliced) or 1 small can of
salmon, sardines or mackerel

3 tablespoons cooked quinoa

A handful of iceberg and
spinach leaves, shredded

1 spring onion, chopped

A few slices of cucumber

1 carrot, grated

$1/4$ turnip or kohlrabi, grated

$1/4$ yellow bell pepper, chopped

A few radishes, sliced

4 cherry tomatoes, halved

Toasted sunflower and pumpkin seeds

Home-made French dressing

Serves 1 person

Method

1. Make a base of the lettuce and spinach leaves in a large Tupperware container.

2. Add the chopped spring onion, cucumber and quinoa. Arrange the grated carrot and turnip, pepper, radishes and tomatoes around the edges of the container. Place the egg or fish in the middle.

3. Sprinkle toasted seeds and drizzle 1 tablespoon of the dressing over the salad.

Tip: Make up a standard French dressing in a bottle or jam jar and keep it ready in the fridge: 1 part apple cider vinegar, 2 parts cold-pressed virgin olive oil, $1/2$ tsp wholegrain mustard, a spot of honey, sea salt, black pepper and herbs to taste.

WAY 24 Know your artichoke

It is easy to get confused about artichokes.

A Jerusalem artichoke is a sweet tasting, knobbly root vegetable and member of the sunflower family. A globe artichoke, on the other hand, is an edible flower bud with silvery-green leaves and, like milk thistle, a member of the thistle family.

Historically, the globe artichoke has been used for liver and gallbladder conditions. It contains excellent levels of fibre, vitamins C and K, folate, magnesium, potassium, calcium, iron and other trace elements. It also contains a number of biologically active phytonutrients. Cynarin is found in the edible base of artichoke leaves and has been used for centuries to increase bile flow and prevent the build-up of sludge and stones in the gallbladder, and help the body to absorb the fat-soluble vitamins A, D, E, and K. The potent flavonoid silymarin is believed to be highly liver protective. Perhaps this is the reason why artichokes have such a high reputation for reducing the symptoms of indigestion and hangovers.

Artichoke leaf extract also shows potential in lowering cholesterol levels, although the evidence is still inconsistent. Use with caution if suffering with gallstones or during pregnancy, as artichokes may worsen bile duct obstruction by increasing bile flow. Globe artichokes look intimidating but are tremendously versatile and can be steamed, boiled, stuffed, chopped, served with sauces or used with quiche, pasta, pizza and risotto dishes.

Jerusalem artichokes can be eaten raw and grated or sliced into salad, boiled and mashed or roasted. These tubers are one of the best sources of inulin, a fructose-based indigestible starch which is associated with a number of health benefits. Inulin can have a potent wind-producing effect, so this artichoke is best introduced in small doses. Inulin can only be digested through bacterial activity and ferments in the large intestine, thereby stimulating the selective growth of beneficial gut bacteria called bifidobacteria* (39), (40).

Bifidobacteria are a group of bacteria in the intestines that help to ward off infection and boost the immune system. These 'friendly' bacteria can be used as a treatment (probiotic) in specific combinations with other bacteria such as the lactobacilli* to prevent children's and traveller's diarrhoea and restore normal intestinal flora following antibiotic therapy. Bifidobacteria may also relieve constipation and help to control the symptoms of ulcerative colitis. Other uses include treating atopic eczema in children and yeast infections (candidiasis). As the inulin from Jerusalem artichokes promotes the growth of these so-called 'friendly' bacteria, it is known as a prebiotic.

SEE ALSO
- **WAY 16: Butter is better** (page 54)

Mashed Jerusalem Artichokes

This is a great, tasty enhancement to ordinary mashed potato.
It is packed with prebiotics which can cause windiness, so start off with small amounts!

Ingredients

250g Jerusalem artichokes

800g potatoes, peeled and cut into chunks
(you can also use sweet potatoes or swede)

50ml milk or milk alternative

2 tbsp butter

Salt and pepper to taste

Small pinch of freshly grated nutmeg

Serves 4-6 people, as a side dish

Method

1. Scrub and peel the potatoes and artichokes, chop into pieces and add to a pot.

2. Bring to the boil, cover and simmer until tender, about 15 minutes, then drain.

3. Add the butter and milk and mash until smooth. Season to taste with salt, pepper and nutmeg.

Try me out

Tip: Jerusalem artichokes are easy to prepare and cook. Globe artichokes less so. To save time, buy ready-to-eat globe artichoke hearts marinated in oil and herbs to accompany bean, potato, grain, pasta or green salads.

WAY 25 Lemon Aid

Lemon trees were first grown in China and India around 4,000 years ago and found their way to Europe with a little help from trade merchants and the Crusaders.

Christopher Columbus was the first to introduce lemons to America, yet was unaware they could prevent scurvy, a vitamin C deficiency disease all-too-common on long sea voyages lacking in fresh food. The British Navy finally made lemon juice mandatory for all sailors in 1795. English ships were required by law to carry sufficient lemon or lime juice for every seaman to have an ounce daily after being at sea for 10 days.

Through the ages, the lemon has been seen as one of the most valuable of all fruit for preserving health. It has been recommended as a cooling drink to relieve thirst and combat fever, to calm anxiety and even used as a cure for obstinate hiccups.

Lemons are an abundant source of vitamin C, as well as bioflavonoids which have strong immune-boosting and anti-oxidant properties and help to strengthen skin and blood vessels. The juice of a lemon, diluted with water, is anti-bacterial and can be used as an emergency disinfectant for minor wounds. It also makes an ideal gargle for sore throats. Heating the mixture and adding a teaspoon of honey and grated ginger produces a classic remedy for coughs and colds. If you want to detox after a period of indulgence, this fruit is the mother of all detox cures. Many people start off their day with a glass of water and a slice of lemon or a splash of freshly-squeezed lemon juice.

Lemon juice mixed with water is often used to ease digestive problems such as the heartburn, indigestion or bloating experienced after heavy meals or eating too quickly. Do not try this folk remedy, however, if suffering from overacidity of the stomach. Although lemons are classified as an acidic fruit, they actually have an alkaline effect on the body as their mineral content forms an alkaline ash as a product of digestion. Lemons are reportedly effective diuretics helping the body eliminate excess fluids, alleviating problems associated with water retention.

If you have any spare lemons, squeeze the juice and freeze in ice cube trays – defrost when needed and add to chilled mineral water or use to flavour food, salad dressings and sauces. It is an excellent preservative, lifts the flavour of vegetable juices and inhibits the discolouration of fresh fruit. When using the rind to flavour and garnish, take care to scrub the lemon thoroughly to remove any fungicide residues and wax before grating.

See also
- **WAY 21: Fish for the brain** (page 64)
- **WAY 38: Turn to turmeric for curcumin cure** (page 98)

Baked Fish with Lemon and Black Pepper

Any white fish can be used, the curry spices and lemon provide valuable nutrients as well as colour and flavour.

Ingredients

3 or 4 favourite white fish fillets

Pinch of sea salt

$^1/_2$ tsp turmeric

1 tsp cumin powder

$^1/_2$ tsp freshly ground black pepper

1 clove garlic finely minced

1 tbsp extra virgin olive oil

2 tsp lemon juice

Serves 2

Method

1. Place fish in a baking dish and sprinkle with salt, turmeric, cumin, black pepper and garlic. Add olive oil. Make sure fish are coated all over, then leave to marinate in the fridge for an hour.

2. Preheat oven to 200°C (400°F). Arrange the fish in a single layer inside the baking dish and cover.

3. Bake for 25 minutes and drizzle with lemon juice just before serving.

Try me out

Tip: By cutting lemons into quarters or slices and then freezing them, you can reduce waste. To clean wooden chopping boards and neutralise odours, regularly rub them with lemon juice, leave overnight and then rinse the next morning.

WAY 26 Mighty mung beans

Whenever you have overindulged or eaten something heavy, allow the humble mung bean to come to your rescue.

Mung beans are tiny, highly nutritious green beans, used for centuries in Chinese and Indian cuisine. They are high in protein, fibre and less likely to make you 'windy' than other beans or pulses. Low in fat and sodium, they contain useful amounts of potassium, magnesium and vitamins B and C.

I first learned about mung beans from my father. He explained that during his childhood in Sri Lanka, breakfast often consisted of mung beans. My grandmother would wash and boil mung beans, add fresh grated coconut, a chilli onion mix and a little lime juice. This would provide an economical, tasty and highly nutritious meal for a family of nine. Mung beans can be sprouted, cooked, or ground into flour. They are versatile and quick to cook and can be prepared in any number of ways. In Indonesia, mung beans are simmered with sugar, ginger and coconut milk to make popular desserts, including ice-cream. They can also be ground into a paste and formed into pancakes, jelly and glass noodles.

In the UK, we are more familiar with sprouted mung beans, eaten as a healthy snack or added to salads, stir-fries and spring-rolls.

Traditionally, mung bean sprouts have been used to reduce fever and heatstroke, and to remove toxic materials. Readily available in supermarkets and healthfood stores, dried mung beans can be added to soups, stews and casseroles instead of lentils. Spices such as ginger, cumin, coriander and turmeric enhance their flavour and improve their digestibility.

The fibre in mung beans is effective for those suffering with a sluggish bowel. The beans also help to control blood sugar, as they provide slow-releasing carbohydrates and protein. Animal studies provide scientific evidence that mung beans improve glucose tolerance and insulin response, without increasing body weight. There is growing interest in the mung bean as a functional food source for diabetics due to its useful glycaemic properties and additional potential to inhibit various diabetic complications, including diabetic nephropathy (41).

In Oriental medicine, fasting on mung bean soup for three days is considered an ideal way of cleansing and detoxifying the body. A short fast with mung bean soup can be done for half a day whenever the body needs a rest after overeating or drinking.

SEE ALSO
- **WAY 7: Fire up your digestion with ginger** (page 30)
- **WAY 22: Garlic is 'as good as ten mothers'** (page 66)
- **WAY 28: Nuts about coconuts** (page 78)

Easy Mung Bean Soup

Some people find mung beans easier to digest than other beans
or lentils. This is a hearty, warming soup that you can freeze in
single portions and enjoy whenever there is little time to prepare a meal.

Ingredients

1 cup dried mung beans
1 onion, chopped
2 cloves garlic, minced
2cm piece of fresh ginger, grated
1 tsp vegetable bouillon powder
3 cups of water
Freshly milled black pepper
1 tbsp creamed coconut (optional)

Serves 4

Method

1. Soak mung beans overnight, wash and drain.

2. Sauté onion, garlic and grated ginger, add mung beans with three times the volume of water and cook for 25 minutes until tender, along with some vegetable stock powder, black pepper, a variety of preferred spices and a little creamed coconut. Add more water if required.

3. Cool a little before blitzing in a blender. Reheat, then serve and enjoy.

Try me out

Tip: To sprout mung beans, soak beans in a jar of clean water for 12 hours, then drain the beans and rinse thoroughly. Return the beans to the jar and cover with a cloth. Rinse and drain the beans once or twice a day. Continue to rinse and drain the sprouts until the sprouts are at least $1/4$ or $1/2$ inch long. Then store in the fridge and use to sprinkle over sandwiches, salads and soups.

WAY 27 No gripes with fennel

In his famous book 'The Complete Herbal' in 1653, the herbalist Nicholas Culpeper pronounced that 'Fennel expels wind, provokes urine, and eases the pains of the stone, and helps to break it.' (25)

Culpeper also recommended fennel tea to nursing mothers to stimulate milk production, and as an effective gripe water for babies. At the time, fennel was already renowned as a versatile aromatic plant – the Ancient Egyptians, Greeks and Romans all used the herb for medicinal and culinary purposes.

Fennel is related to parsley, carrots, coriander and dill, and is similar in looks and texture to celery. Native to the Mediterranean region, it is commonly added raw to salads or can be lightly cooked or roasted, providing a distinctive aniseed flavour to dishes. Fennel is popular served with fish. The bulb, stalk, leaves and seeds of the plant are all edible. The leaves can be used to flavour virgin olive oil and its seeds used to flavour ice cream and liqueurs.

Fennel has a long tradition of supporting digestive health. In India, fennel seeds are chewed after meals to freshen the breath. The seeds help to stimulate the production of gastric juices which improves the entire process of digestion and absorption. Fennel tea is often recommended to treat heartburn and colic as well as upper respiratory infections. Large amounts of fennel should be avoided during pregnancy, however, as its mild oestrogenic-like qualities may stimulate contractions.

Fennel contains a number of valuable phytonutrients, including the flavonoids rutin and quercitin. Most interesting, however, are its volatile oils. Anethole, a primary component in fennel oil is involved in blocking an intercellular signalling system associated with inflammation. Researchers propose that by shutting down the signalling system, anethole in fennel may prevent the activation of cellular responses that can alter genes and trigger off inflammation (43).

Add thinly sliced fennel to sandwiches as an alternative topping. Or use as a tasty side-dish, cutting fennel bulbs into quarters and gently braising them in melted butter with a little chicken or vegetable stock.

Fresh fennel should be stored in the fridge and keeps fresh for about four days. Dried fennel seeds should also be stored in an airtight container in the fridge where they will keep for at least six months. According to Master Culpeper 'a decoction of the leaves and root is good for serpent bites, and to neutralize vegetable poison, as mushrooms'. So take note, fennel is a handy ingredient to have in your kitchen!

SEE ALSO
- **WAY 16: Butter is better** (page 54)
- **WAY 19: Chicken soup for the soul and the nose** (page 62)
- **WAY 31: Parsley, the potent free radical fighter** (page 84)

Fennel Pea Risotto

Refrigerate if you have any leftover risotto and
use as a tasty filler in your salad tomorrow.

Ingredients

1 tbsp extra-virgin olive oil or ghee
1 red onion, finely chopped
1 bulb fennel, diced
1 clove garlic, minced
1 cup arborio (paella) rice
650ml vegetable bouillon or chicken stock
1 cup frozen or fresh peas
2 tbsp chopped fresh parsley
Sea salt and black pepper

Serves 4

Method

1. Heat the oil or ghee in a large saucepan
   over medium heat and gently cook the
   onion, fennel and garlic until softened.
2. Add the rice, stirring to coat and toast
   the grains. Begin adding the broth
   mixture, 1 cup (125 ml) at a time, stirring
   after each addition until most of the
   liquid is absorbed before adding more.
   The whole process should take about
   20 minutes.
3. Stir in the peas,
   seasoning and any
   remaining broth and
   cook until the peas
   are tender, about 3
   minutes, then sprinkle
   the parsley over the rice and serve.

Tip: Fennel is particularly tasty when combined with oily fish such as mackerel.
Stuff the fish with its leaves and add sliced fennel to the water used for poaching
the fish.

28 Nuts about coconuts

What plant provides milk, flesh, sugar, oil and acts as its own dish and cup? A coconut, of course, which isn't botanically speaking a nut at all, but the largest known seed.

Even its husk can be used as fuel, or to make brushes and fishing nets. In the ancient Indian language of Sanskrit the coconut is described as the 'tree which gives all that is necessary for living'.

The watery liquid inside a young coconut is the best natural sports drink you can find, containing valuable nutrients and electrolytes, salts and sugars. Creamy coconut milk is made by squeezing grated coconut flesh with hot water. The top layer of the milk can be skimmed off and used as coconut cream.

Polynesian and Indian women use coconut oil to soften skin and hair and as protection from the sun (44). For silky smooth hair, apply a small amount of the pure oil onto your hair before going to bed and wash it out the next morning.

People in the tropics have used coconut oil in their diet for thousands of years and attribute their lower incidence of some diseases to its nutritional benefits. Although around 92% of coconut fat is saturated fat, the saturated fat from tropical oils differs from animal fat

associated with heart disease (45). Over 50% of the fats in coconut are medium-chain triglycerides. These have unique therapeutic benefits for dieters and athletes as they are immediately converted into energy rather than stored as fat (46).

Coldpressed virgin coconut oil (VCO) made from fresh coconut kernels does not contain trans fats, which are now considered more harmful than saturated fats. There is even evidence that VCO helps to maintain normal levels of cholesterol and other lipids (47). It is a rich source of lauric acid which is found naturally in human breast milk. Lauric acid is converted into the potent anti-microbial agent monolaurin by the body (48).

Coconut oil can be used as a spread or added to food and drink. Unlike most other oils, coconut oil remains relatively stable when heated and is preferable for cooking, frying and baking. It can be safely heated up to temperatures of 190°C (375°F).

Coconut oil has a long shelf life and is ideally stored in a cool, dark place. Naturally solid at room temperature, it will melt in hot weather or if you put the tub in hot water. Ensure your supply has not been hydrogenated, bleached, deodorised and is as organic as the beautiful tree from which it was created.

SEE ALSO
• **WAY 22: Garlic is 'as good as ten mothers'** (page 66)

Tip: To boost your immune system include 2 tbsp of VCO per day in food or drinks. Eat it straight from the spoon, add to shakes and smoothies, or mix with warm water or tea. Or simply grate over salads, add to sauces or use in baking.

Coconut Potato Chips

Coconut oil (or butter) is one of the safest and healthiest
cooking oils and is now also available without the coconut taste and aroma.

Ingredients

4–5 large organic potatoes
A few cloves garlic, minced
3 tbsp virgin coconut oil
1 tbsp tamari soy sauce
2 tsp smoked paprika spice

Serves 4

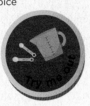

Method

1. Preheat oven to 180°C (350°F).
   Melt the coconut oil in the oven in
   a large baking tray.
2. Wash potatoes well, then cut into
   thick slices but do not peel them.
   Cut the slices into chips and place
   onto baking tray.
3. Mix with chopped garlic and coat
   well with the melted coconut oil
   and soy sauce before baking. Sprinkle
   with paprika or other preferred herbs
   or spices.
4. Check chips after 20 minutes and turn.
   Cook for a further 15 minutes, or until
   tender but crunchy.

WAY 29 Olives and the Mediterranean diet

Enjoyed by people living in Spain, Portugal, France, Italy, Greece and Cyprus, the Mediterranean diet is associated with wide-ranging health benefits and a decreased risk of Type 2 diabetes, obesity, heart disease, cancer and Alzheimer's Disease.

The Mediterranean diet relies on plant-based foods such as fruits and vegetables, wholegrains, legumes, nuts and fish, moderate red wine consumption and little red meat.

One of the main ingredients of the Mediterranean diet is olive oil, and in ancient times, it was considered as valuable as gold. Olive oil is pressed from the flesh of whole ripe olives, the fruits of the tree. The olive tree has been cultivated for over 7,000 years and its oil has been used as a nutritious food, medicine and beauty treatment (49). 'Extra virgin' olive oil is produced from the first pressing of the olives, and 'virgin' olive oil from the second pressing. If an olive oil is not labelled 'virgin', it has been filtered, refined and possibly heated and deodorised, consequently suffering nutrient losses and other changes.

Olives vary in colour, size, shape, flavour and chemical composition. They cannot be eaten straight from the tree due to their bitter flavour, and to make them more palatable, they are fermented or cured with lye or brine. Olives are exceptionally rich in oleic acid, a monounsaturated fat* that may help reduce the amount of the more harmful low-density lipoprotein (LDL) cholesterol in the blood.

Black olives are also rich in vitamin E, iron and a number of phenolic compounds which have anti-inflammatory and anti-oxidant properties.

Apart from being nourishing and economical, this way of eating is also truly delicious. The following Mediterranean diet principles can easily be followed at home:

- Avoid processed, refined foods and look for seasonal, locally grown fruit and vegetables. Aim to make plant foods (fruit, vegetables, nuts, beans, wholegrains) the main ingredients at mealtimes.
- Eat fish and seafood at least twice a week, poultry once a week and red meat only a few times a month.
- Staple foods such as rice, wholegrain bread, potatoes, pasta or couscous are always accompanied by plenty of vegetables.
- Drizzle vegetables and fresh salads with olive oil. The consumption of tomatoes with olive oil is particularly beneficial. Olive oil improves the absorption and anti-oxidant activity of lycopene, the red pigment in tomatoes.
- To flavour dishes, use garlic, onions and bell peppers and plenty of fresh or dried herbs such as thyme, basil and oregano.
- For snacks, eat fresh or dried fruit with nuts. Avoid crisps and sweets.
- The anti-oxidant resveratrol, produced by grapes in response to stress, has been identified as a key ingredient in red wine. Wine should be consumed in moderation and at mealtimes.

SEE ALSO
- **WAY 14: Apple cider vinegar, an extraordinary nutritional drink** (page 50)
- **WAY 30: Oregano, joy of the mountains** (page 82)

Traditional Greek Salad

An all-time classic, this mouth-watering Greek summer salad
can be served as a side dish or as a light meal on its own.

Ingredients

3 ripe tomatoes, chopped
1 cucumber, chopped
1 small red onion, chopped
16 pitted black olives, halved
85g feta cheese, cut into chunks
1 clove garlic, minced
1 tsp dried oregano
Sea salt and pepper to taste
1 $^1/_2$ tbsp lemon juice or apple cider vinegar
3 tbsp Greek extra virgin olive oil

Serves 4–6

Method

1. Place the olive oil, lemon juice (or vinegar), garlic, oregano, salt and pepper in a small jar with a screw-top lid and shake well.
2. Combine all other ingredients in a large bowl, pour the dressing over the salad and mix gently.

Try me out

Tip: Wash olives well before eating as they are packaged in brine and are therefore high in salt.

30

Oregano, joy of the mountains

One of my favourite herbs is oregano, the herb more commonly known as an aromatic flavouring for Mediterranean dishes.

Oregano is closely related to marjoram and is usually found sprinkled over pizzas or scrambled eggs. Through the ages it has been added to German sausages, English herbal snuffs, even French soaps and pomades. Before the discovery of hops, beer was flavoured with oregano and, as it effectively prevents the growth of microbes, the herb was used as a natural preservative.

Oregano grows wild in the Greek mountains and legend has it that the Greek goddess Aphrodite created its fragrance for the peace and well-being of mankind. Maybe every household should keep a jar handy! The ancient Greeks used it internally and externally for a variety of conditions. Poultices were made from the leaves to treat sores and aching muscles and it was a popular antidote to the poison from snakes and scorpions. In Europe, oregano has traditionally been used to treat respiratory problems such as coughs, bronchitis and sinusitis. A powerful expectorant, it helps to break up mucous in the respiratory tract.

The health benefits of oregano are mainly due to the highly active compounds of its essential oil. The most important ingredients in the oil are carvacrol and thymol which have potent antimicrobial, antiviral and antifungal properties. An increasing amount of evidence supports the claims that oregano oil is an effective therapeutic agent for Candida albicans, E. coli, salmonella, Staphylococcus, influenza and some pneumonia-causing bugs. It has also been used to treat intestinal parasites.

Reports suggest that oregano may ease flatulence and other digestive complaints. In order to settle the stomach or soothe a cough, you can make a spicy tea by steeping one to two teaspoons of fresh or dried oregano in a cup of boiling water for ten minutes. The herb is particularly effective for sinus infections which are often due to an underlying fungal problem. Although modern antibiotics work fast and effectively, if used on a recurring basis they cause bacterial imbalance in the GI tract which may trigger off further fungal overgrowth and make the situation worse in the long run.

Before taking the potent oil of oregano, consult a herbal, nutritional or medical practitioner to ensure the correct dosage which should be tailored to the individual person and complaint. Pregnant women can safely use the herb as a seasoning but should avoid consuming large amounts of oregano oil as it may promote menstruation. The name oregano is derived from the Greek and means 'Joy of the Mountains'. It certainly deserves more credit than for being known merely as a culinary spice.

SEE ALSO
- **WAY 9: Most definately go to work on an egg** (page 34)
- **WAY 22: Garlic is 'as good as ten mothers'** (page 66)

Mama's Meat Loaf with Oregano

Meatloaf can be served hot with new potatoes and vegetables,
or cut into slices when cold for sandwiches and lunchboxes.

Ingredients

$1/2$ pound minced beef
$1/2$ pound minced pork
2 eggs, lightly beaten
1 cup breadcrumbs
2 large cloves of garlic, minced
1 large onion, chopped
$1/4$ cup diced green bell pepper
1 tsp dried oregano
Freshly ground pepper to taste
1 tbsp Worcester sauce
1 tsp mustard
1 tsp dried vegetable bouillon
4 tbsp tomato paste

Serves 8

Method

1. Combine beef, pork, eggs, breadcrumbs, garlic, onion, green pepper, oregano, bouillon, pepper, Worcester sauce, mustard and 2 tbsp tomato paste in a large bowl.
2. Mix thoroughly with your (clean) hands.
3. Pack into a greased loaf tin. Cover with the remaining 2 tbsp tomato paste.
4. Bake for 1 hour and 15 minutes at 180°C (350°F) in a preheated oven.
5. Let meatloaf rest for 15 minutes before sprinkling with dried or fresh oregano and cutting to serve.

Tip: When cooking or baking with oregano, remember to add it in the last few minutes as it can taste bitter if overcooked and loses its valuable antibacterial qualities. Dried oregano quickly loses its pungency and needs to be replaced regularly.

WAY 31

Parsley, the potent free radical fighter

All too familiar as a simple plate garnish, parsley is often overlooked in favour of more exotic sounding herbs, but it contains far too many health benefits to be ignored for long.

Take your time to rediscover this herb in a different way. Rather than imagining a solitary dry sprig garnished on top of a lamb chop, think of finely chopped parsley and garlic drizzled over roast potatoes, or added at the end of cooking time to enhance sauces, soups and vegetables.

Parsley is a member of the celery and carrot family and there are two main types: flat leaf or curly. Apart from its culinary talents, parsley has a variety of medicinal uses and boasts a long and distinguished history. The Ancient Greeks crowned their athletes with wreaths of parsley and the Romans made parsley garlands for banquets in order to counteract strong odours.

Traditionally used as a diuretic to support the urinary system, parsley encourages the elimination of water from the body. It has also been used to offer some relief from the painful condition gout to aid the excretion of uric acid, a waste product left over from normal chemical processes in the body. An abnormal build-up of uric acid may cause gout. Other applications have included improving liver and digestive function, for example as a hangover 'cure' or to reduce gas and colic. Over the ages, the herb has also been used to treat menstrual disorders due to its volatile oils apiol and myristicin which are believed to stimulate the uterus. For this reason, large amounts should be avoided during pregnancy, or if suffering from kidney disease.

Parsley is packed with nutrients, especially vitamins A, C and K. The flavonoid apigenin found in parsley is currently being investigated for its potential to delay the onset of some forms of breast cancer (50). Recently there has been interest in parsley's high glutathione content. Glutathione is a less well known, but important anti-oxidant present in many fruits and vegetables, especially parsley, broccoli and spinach. Glutathione is the most important anti-oxidant in the interior of the human cell and either works on its own or teams up with the mineral selenium. Together they form an important anti-oxidant enzyme, glutathione peroxidase, which appears to protect cell membranes from damage by reactive oxygen species, also known as free radicals.

Free radicals are highly reactive, unstable molecules produced in the body by normal biochemical processes and by external factors such as smoking, excess alcohol, over-exercising, pollution or radiation. In excess, they contribute to molecular damage and may be a factor in aging and disease. Anti-oxidants help to neutralize free radicals. As a high percentage of glutathione is lost during cooking and processing, it is best absorbed from raw food.

Parsley is a tasty and convenient source and no elaborate herb garden is required, a balcony or sunny window spot will do nicely.

SEE ALSO
- **WAY 2: Almonds, the all-rounders** (page 20)
- **WAY 29: Olives and the Mediterranean diet** (page 80)

Parsley Pesto with Goat's Cheese

If you have a passion for pesto, mix it with pasta or
serve with sliced tomatoes and baked potatoes.

Ingredients

5 tbsp extra virgin olive oil
4 level tbsp freshly chopped parsley
$1/2$ cup (50g) walnuts, chopped
Sea salt and freshly ground black pepper
2 x 100g mature round goat's cheese

Serve 2

Method

1. To make the pesto, combine the olive oil,
   chopped parsley, walnuts and seasoning
   in a food processor or blender and
   process until smooth.
2. Cut the goat's cheeses in half widthways
   and place in mini gratin dishes, or on foil
   with the cut surface facing upwards.
3. Place under a hot grill until the cheese
   turns golden and just
   starts to melt.
4. Spoon some of the
   pesto over the cheese.
   Serve immediately
   with a green leafy
   salad and grilled
   tomatoes.

Tip: Chew on a sprig of parsley to freshen up your breath after consuming onions,
garlic, alcohol or nicotine (but check your teeth afterwards!).

32

Pick your perfect pumpkin

Food is the most conventional form of medicine; it used to be regarded as both nourishment and treatment. So it is with the magnificent pumpkin and its seeds.

Pumpkins belong to the gourd family which includes the marrow, cucumber and squash. They were one of the crops first cultivated by Native American Indians who liked to eat pumpkin pieces after roasting them over open fires.

The Pilgrims learned the value of pumpkins from the Indians and created pumpkin soup, pumpkin beer and pumpkin pie. Pumpkins are incredibly versatile, easy to digest and the nutty-tasting flesh is a useful source of vitamin E and beta-carotene. They also contain calcium, magnesium, potassium and iron. Europeans were introduced to pumpkins when explorers returned from the New World with their new seeds.

The name 'squash' comes from a tribal Indian word 'askutasquash' meaning 'something eaten raw'. Nothing went to waste: they were consumed uncooked, or baked in hot ashes and eaten with honey or maple syrup; the seeds were toasted or ground into a paste; and the hard outer rinds were used as bowls and storage jars.

Popular modern varieties apart from pumpkin include butternut, acorn, kabocha and spaghetti squash. They make cheap and nourishing additions to a meal and can be kept through the winter months without spoiling as their thick, hard skins protect flavour and texture. Store them in a cool, dry place away from direct sun, but not in plastic bags, as this will encourage them to rot.

Butternut is one of the most popular squash and the longer it is stored, the sweeter it tastes. Pear shaped, with a deep orange-coloured flesh, butternut has a mild, nutty flavour and is an excellent source of alpha- and beta-carotene, as well as many other vitamins and minerals, helping to boost our beleaguered immune systems over the winter months. Technically a squash is a fruit, but is frequently treated like a vegetable. You can consume it in many different ways; an all-time favourite is pumpkin pie (butternut squash or acorn can also be used and frozen if you have leftovers). Baking squash is easy, preserves its nutrients and intensifies its flavours.

Like the Native American Indians, you can also eat your squash raw by using a cheese grater and mixing it into a salad. If you prefer squash cooked, simply cut one into chunks, peel off the rind with a sharp knife, steam and mash with a little butter. Or add to pancake batter, stews, soups and curries. Squash adds moisture, colour and sweetness to breads, pies and cakes. When cooked and pureed, it is a delicious, nutritious food for young children.

SEE ALSO
- **WAY 29: Olives and the Mediterranean diet** (page 80)
- **WAY 47: Seeds: all good things come in small packages** (page 122)

Baked Butternut Squash

Turn the seeds from your butternut squash into a healthy snack:
wash and pat the seeds dry, gently toss in olive oil and sprinkle with salt.
Roast in the oven for about an hour or pop them into
the dehydrater if you prefer them raw.

Ingredients

1 butternut squash
Olive oil for drizzling
2 tbsp butter
Sea salt and freshly ground black pepper
Fresh or dried thyme

Serve 4

Try me out

Method

1. Preheat oven to 180°C (350°F).
2. Cut butternut squash in half lengthwise and scoop out the seeds with a spoon.
3. Place the halves cut side up on a baking sheet. Drizzle the olive oil over the top and dot with the butter. Season to taste with salt and freshly ground black pepper, then sprinkle with thyme.
4. Roast in the oven for around 45 minutes, or until the squash is tender.

Tip: Buy pumpkins and winter squashes from farms or farmers' markets in autumn. Store in a cool, dry, dark place (shed/garage/loft) on cloth, straw or cardboard. Place in a well-ventilated position at a temperature under 15°C (60°F) and no colder than 10°C (50°F). Most pumpkin varieties will store for at least 3 months.

WAY 33

Provide each day a healthy bread

Paleolithic humans were long considered predominantly carnivorous. However, grain residues have been discovered on grinding stones at different archaeological sites, suggesting that starchy grains were already being processed 30,000 years ago (51).

The theory is that our hunter–gatherer ancestors began grinding wild grains and mixing the resultant 'flour' with water into a thick paste. The mixture was formed into flatbreads, then dried in the sun or cooked on hot stones, creating a primitive type of bread.

Since then, various cultures have refined the art of bread baking. The Ancient Egyptians used closed ovens and were the first to experiment with yeast, producing a raised loaf. Now, we see large automated baking units and faster industrial methods that satisfy demand and increase productivity. Modern food technology has managed to perfect the art of light-textured 'cotton-wool' bread which can be stacked easily and stored for long periods of time.

If we look at the food labels, we see our convenience bread of today bears no resemblance to the wholefood of our ancestors. Common ingredients found in the soft, squishy slices include bread improvers, enzymes, raising agents, preservatives, emulsifiers, stabilisers and partially hydrogenated oils. As for brown bread, it may be white bread disguised with caramel colouring.

Apart from large amounts of added chemicals, flours have been so heavily refined that over half the nutrients and most of the fibre have been removed. Refined flours coat and clog the intestines, interfering with the rhythm and proper functioning of the digestive tract. Stagnation of waste leads to the development of undesirable micro-organisms which may promote disease or intolerances. Some people may simply be affected by the ingredients bread contains, others by the way in which their bread has been produced.

Increasingly, bread companies and bakeries are introducing nutritious whole grain products. Master bakers believe the length of time it takes for the dough to ripen and rise is of prime importance. There are traditional bakeries that have gone back to basics using freshly milled organic grains and a traditional fermentation process with natural enzymes rather than added yeast or synthetic chemicals. Different breads can be baked, depending on the needs and preferences of the individual: some varieties contain freshly sprouted grains, some are wheat- and gluten-free and suitable for those suffering with food intolerances. The slow mixing, long fermentation and proving process makes the bread more digestible and allows it to develop in taste and vitality, a preferable alternative to both prehistoric and modern supermarket varieties!

SEE ALSO

- **WAY 16: Butter is better** (page 54)
- **WAY 26: Mighty mung beans** (page 74)
- **WAY 47: Seeds: all good things come in small packages** (page 122)

My Favourite Sandwich

This is also good with other seed and nut butters,
including pumpkin seed butter or cashew nut butter.

Ingredients

Artisan bread (wheat, rice, buckwheat,
linseed, quinoa, pea, rye, spelt or
essene bread) (52)
Butter for spreading
Tahini (sesame paste)
Fresh mung bean sprouts, washed

*Serves as many as your bread,
tahini and mung beans supply allows!*

Method

1. Spread a slice of artisan bread with
   butter and tahini and sprinkle with
   a thick layer of mung bean sprouts.
2. Eat!

Tip: Find a quality bread containing pure ingredients without improvers, enzymes,
excess salt, sugar and yeast. Buy in bulk, slice and freeze in small batches. Take out
individual slices and toast when required.

WAY 34

Quinoa, an old food for the future

There is an increasing interest in alternatives to gluten-containing grains (wheat, rye and barley) due to the rising incidence of Coeliac Disease and gluten sensitivity.

Coeliac Disease is an autoimmune disorder triggered when gluten is ingested and the body starts producing antibodies that attack its own tissues. Common symptoms include extreme fatigue, abdominal pain, bloating, diarrhoea, anaemia and weight loss. Some people may also experience depression, mouth ulcers and dermatitis.

Modern wheat is very high in gluten and our consumption of wheat has risen to such an extent that many people are eating it three times a day or more. Wheat is found in bread, biscuits, cakes, cereals, pastry and is an added ingredient in many processed foods. Those who do not suffer from Coeliac Disease but also experience symptoms when eating gluten-containing products, are generally defined as gluten sensitive.

Not surprisingly, interest is growing in alternatives to wheat and sustainable protein-rich foods of plant origin. Spotlight on quinoa (pronounced 'keenwa'), an ancient food from high in the South American Andes which boasts a higher nutritional value than most traditional cereals (53). It thrives in harsh conditions of 10,000 feet, low rainfall, poor soil and freezing temperatures and has been cultivated in the Andean region for 7,000 years.

Long before the arrival of the Spanish conquistadors, the Inca civilisation revered quinoa as sacred because of its exceptional nutritional profile. The 'Mother Grain' contains all nine essential amino acids and is therefore higher in protein than many other cereals. It is rich in fibre and an excellent source of calcium, phosphorus, iron and vitamins E and B. No wonder then, that the Incas were famous for their strength and high-altitude climbing.

Quinoa is not technically a cereal grain but the seed of a fruit. It resembles millet in appearance and the most common varieties are golden or red. When cooked, quinoa has a delicious nutty taste, suitable for sweet and savoury dishes. Unlike many other grains, it is easy to digest and takes just 10–15 minutes to prepare. Rinse well in a fine-mesh strainer, drain and bring to boil in a saucepan (use two cups of water for every cup of quinoa), then reduce to simmer and cook until soft and you can see the germ ring on the outer edge of the seed. Use plain water for cooking or add vegetable or meat stock. Quinoa is a delicious, practical alternative to rice, pasta or potatoes. Use it in soups, casseroles, stir-fries – or even cold in shakes, puddings or sprinkled over salads.

You can buy quinoa in your local health food shop or supermarket ready to cook, or as flour, pasta or breakfast flakes. Not bad for the humble all-rounder first cultivated thousands of years ago.

SEE ALSO
- **WAY 2: Almonds, the all-rounders** (page 20)
- **WAY 16: Butter is better** (page 54)
- **WAY 47: Seeds: all good things come in small packages** (page 122)

Quinoa Nut Salad

Quinoa stores well in the fridge for up to four days, so make a
little more than required and use the leftovers to invent tasty stir-fries and salads.

Ingredients

1 cup quinoa, well washed

2 cups water

1 tbsp butter or ghee

2 cloves garlic, crushed

1 large courgette, chopped

1 onion, chopped

1 red bell pepper, chopped

100g cashews

100g walnut pieces

50g raisins

25g pumpkin seeds

*Makes 3 or 4 portions as a main
meal and can also be eaten cold*

Method

1. Boil two cups water in a saucepan, add quinoa and simmer with the lid on for 12–14 minutes. Drain and rinse well.

2. Meanwhile, gently sauté onions, pepper and courgette with garlic in butter or ghee until softened.

3. Add the cooked quinoa and the nuts, seeds and fruit. Mix well and allow to heat through. Season to taste.

Try me out

Tip: To deter pests, quinoa seeds are coated with saponins, plant compounds that produce a frothy, soap-like effect when mixed with water. Saponins are generally rinsed off by manufacturers, but it is best to rinse the seeds again thoroughly under cold running water before cooking, lightly rubbing them with your fingers to get rid of any powdery residue.

WAY 35

Sauerkraut, the art of preserving food

Growing awareness that good nutrition is the basis for good health is creating a market for simple, traditional foods that haven't been factory processed or dosed with man-made chemicals.

At the same time there is an interest in rediscovering ancient methods of cooking and preserving foods. How did mankind cope before the invention of fridge freezers and sell-by-dates?

An ideal method of preserving vegetables is by lactic-acid fermentation. This process, in which sugars are converted to lactic acid, produces a sour taste and improves the food's microbiological stability. Fermented vegetables have always been important sources of nourishment. Archaeologists have discovered that fermented plant foods were first consumed by prehistoric hunter-gatherers. One of the most well-known is salted, fermented cabbage, known as sauerkraut. The Chinese have been fermenting cabbage since 200 BC, and used sauerkraut juice as a cure for common ailments. The Romans carried barrels of sauerkraut to prevent intestinal infections on long excursions, and Genghis Khan is said to have transported pickled cabbage to Europe in the 13th century.

Apart from its deliciously tangy flavour, sauerkraut offers remarkable health benefits, such as improving digestion. The fibre and lactic acid bacteria facilitate the breakdown of proteins and promote the growth of healthy bowel flora, protecting against constipation and diseases of the digestive tract. Sauerkraut is fibre-rich, low in calories and high in minerals and vitamin C. Many sailors died from scurvy caused by a lack of vitamin C in their diets until, in the 18th century, the explorer Captain James Cook discovered sauerkraut was an effective remedy for the disease. On his voyages around the world he insisted that his crew ate sauerkraut, no doubt saving countless lives.

More recently, Finnish researchers reported in the *Journal of Agricultural and Food Chemistry* that during the fermentation process, enzymes are released, degrading the cabbage into anti-carcinogenic compounds called isothiocyanates. An association between cabbage and sauerkraut consumption and a lower risk of breast cancer has been observed in Polish immigrants living in the US. Polish women who, as teenagers, ate at least three servings a week of raw or lightly-cooked cabbage and sauerkraut, had a significantly reduced risk of breast cancer later in life compared to those who only ate one serving per week (54).

Sauerkraut contains the healthy bacterial strain Lactobacillus plantarum which has significant immune boosting properties (55). Scientists are currently investigating different starter cultures to improve the fermentation process and further increase health benefits. Commercially available fermented products are generally pasteurized and lack friendly bacterial cultures and may contain vinegar to make the sauerkraut appear fermented. To experience the delicious taste and health benefits of real sauerkraut, you may have to resort to making it yourself, just like our hardy ancestors.

SEE ALSO
- **WAY 15: Broccoli and the astonishing crucifers** (page 52)

Home-made Sauerkraut Recipe

Fermented cabbage or other cultured vegetables are usually ready within 4 to 7 days, although the longer they ferment, the more probiotic support they provide. Sauerkraut is excellent accompanied with a main meal or added to sandwiches, salads and soups (towards the end of cooking).

Ingredients

1 shredded cabbage
10 juniper berries
1 tsp caraway seeds
1–2 tsp non-iodized pickling salt
1 cup of filtered water mixed with 1 tsp non-iodized salt

Try me out

Makes about 4 cups (approximately 1 ltr)

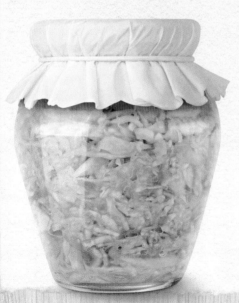

Method

1. In a sterile glass jar or stoneware crock, mix cabbage, juniper berries, caraway seeds and salt. Packing a bit into the jar at a time and pressing down hard with a wooden mallet helps force water out of the cabbage. The salt draws juice out of the cabbage and the resulting 'brine' allows the cabbage to ferment gently.

2. Add filtered, or non-chlorinated, salty water (1 teaspoon salt per cup of warm water) up to the rim of the jar.

3. Using a small plate (or lid) about 1cm smaller in diameter than your container and a weight (a large stone will do), weigh down the cabbage to keep it under the liquid and cap loosely with a lid. Place the jar on a tray to catch overflowing juices.

4. Keep jar between 60°F to 70°F for one to three weeks. The fermentation process will take longer in cooler weather or a cooler room. Check container regularly and top off with salty water if level falls below rim. When ready, skim any (harmless) mould from the top, close jar tightly and store in the fridge.

Tip: To promote optimal digestion and assimilation of nutrients, eat a little sauerkraut before or with every meal, especially later in the day with heavier meals. If you have digestive problems drink a few tablespoons of sauerkraut juice daily.

WAY 36

Spinach, iron and muscle strength

Popeye, the popular cartoon character, ate mounds of spinach thinking it contained plenty of iron to make him strong.

As it turns out, spinach contains high levels of oxalates which bind to the iron, making the mineral more difficult to absorb. It also is not necessarily true that the higher your iron intake, the stronger you become. Increasing iron intake only makes you feel stronger if you are iron deficient in the first place.

Iron is part of haemoglobin, the red pigment in the blood, which carries oxygen to all the cells around the body. Iron-deficiency anaemia results in a decrease in the amount of oxygen the blood is able to carry. Symptoms include unusual fatigue, lack of concentration, dizziness and palpitations. More advanced symptoms can be headaches, a sore or swollen tongue, pale skin and 'restless' legs.

A lack of iron may be due dietary deficiencies or conditions that cause blood loss such as heavy menstruation, piles, ulcers or gastrointestinal bleeding. Pregnant women, people with gluten intolerance, children or adolescents during a growth spurt, or those who simply don't produce enough gastric acid for proper digestion may be at risk of iron deficiency. It is important to get a medical diagnosis and to be aware that there could be many different reasons for fatigue, not just iron deficiency. Apart from iron, the body requires vitamin B12 and folic acid to produce red blood cells. If there is a lack of any of these, anaemia may develop.

The most absorbable form of iron is called 'heme' iron and good sources are red meat, eggs, the dark meat of poultry and oily fish like sardines. 'Non-heme' iron is less well absorbed and found in fortified cereals, beans, nuts, seeds, dried fruit and dark green vegetables like spinach. Vegetarians who do not replace meat with iron-rich foods may be low in the mineral. The body will absorb more iron if it is combined with vitamin C-containing foods such as tomatoes, bell peppers, asparagus, green cabbage, peas or squash.

Popeye was not entirely misguided about spinach making him stronger. A Swedish study has found that spinach contains nitrates which boost the production of two key proteins in muscles involved with calcium and muscle contractions, making them stronger and more efficient. Although the study was done in mice and needs to be replicated in humans, Popeye seems to have had the right idea (56). Spinach is also an excellent source of folate, potassium and magnesium and is rich in carotenoids.

Spinach and other dark green leafy vegetables such as kale, chard and spring greens provide significant health benefits and should be eaten very regularly. Packed with fibre along with vitamins, minerals and potent anti-oxidant compounds, these super veggies help protect against cellular damage implicated in a large number of degenerative conditions – the darker the leaves, the better.

SEE ALSO

- **WAY 22: Garlic is 'as good as ten mothers'** (page 66)
- **WAY 25: Lemon Aid** (page 72)
- **WAY 29: Olives and the Mediterranean diet** (page 80)

Spinach and Tomato Salad

Perfect for lunch with a sliced hard-boiled
egg or as a side salad for your evening meal.

Ingredients

250g cherry tomatoes, halved
A handful of pitted black olives, halved
100g baby spinach leaves, washed
$1/2$ red onion, finely sliced
1 tbsp fresh basil leaves, chopped
1 tbsp lemon juice
1 tbsp olive oil
Salt and pepper to taste

Serves 3-4

Method

1. Combine the tomatoes, olives, spinach
   leaves and onion in a bowl.
2. Make the dressing by adding the basil,
   lemon juice, olive oil and seasoning to
   a screw top jar and
   shaking well. Just
   before serving,
   drizzle over salad.

Try me out

Tip: Cooking spinach reduces its vitamin levels but boosts the bioavailability of its carotenoids. You can get the best out of spinach by lightly steaming the vegetable to accompany a main meal, as well as enjoying fresh spinach leaves raw in salads or sandwiches.

37

The sweetness of sweet potato

Sweet potatoes are root vegetables and should not be confused with ordinary spuds, which are tubers rather than roots.

Native to South and Central America, they were recorded by early Spanish explorers and called 'batatas' by the American Indians.

There are many different varieties of sweet potato, the most commonly known are the sweet orange-fleshed ones and the creamy-coloured drier types. An excellent source of fibre if eaten along with their skins, they are low in fat and supply protein, potassium, calcium and the vitamins C and E. The reddish sweet potatoes are unusually high in powerful anti-oxidants called carotenoids.

Carotenoids are found in red, yellow, orange and green leafy vegetables. The carotenoid family has over 600 members and the most commonly known are beta- and alpha-carotene (sweet potato, carrots), lycopene (tomatoes), lutein (greens), zeaxanthin (corn) and capsanthin (paprika). Carotenoid pigments shield plants from the powerful energy of sunlight and help protect us against sunburn.

The human body is able to convert beta-carotene into the important fat-soluble vitamin A needed for vision, the immune response and to strengthen the skin, bones and internal membranes. Sweet potatoes, with their high carotene content, are therefore an ideal choice. If you eat a little fat (olive oil, butter) with your sweet potato, you significantly increase your uptake of beta-carotene. Some people, however, are less able to absorb beta-carotene

adequately or possess a genetic variability preventing them from efficiently converting it into the active form of vitamin A and still require dietary sources of vitamin A such as fish, cod liver oil, eggs, meat and butter (57).

Sweet potatoes are high in complex carbohydrates, which keep you full for longer than simple carbohydrates such as white potatoes. Jamaican research has found that different methods of preparing sweet potatoes influence their glycaemic index* (GI), a measure of the effects of carbohydrates on blood sugar levels. Tubers processed by boiling had the lowest GI while those roasted and baked had a significantly higher GI (58). Consumption of boiled or steamed sweet potatoes may therefore minimize the risk of blood glucose spikes after meals. Excess consumption of high GI foods may lead to chronically elevated levels of insulin, insulin resistance and weight gain, which are associated with chronic diseases such as Type 2 diabetes and cardiovascular disease.

What do you do with sweet potatoes? Anything and everything because they are so versatile and tasty. If in a hurry, grate some raw over your salad. Or you can rub a little oil on them and bake them in the oven for 30–40 minutes. Or steam them and add a little butter before serving. Once cooked and mashed, they make great desserts. Ever tried Sweet Potato Pie or Pudding? Children love sweet potato bread and muffins or smoothies containing sweet potatoes, orange juice and yoghurt.

SEE ALSO

- **WAY 22: Garlic is 'as good as ten mothers'** (page 66)
- **WAY 29: Olives and the Mediterranean diet** (page 80)

Roasted Vegetables

Scrumptious and succulent as a side dish to a main meal,
or allow to cool and combine with rice or quinoa to make a glorious roast veggie salad.

Ingredients

2 red onions, thickly sliced
1 sweet potato, diced
2 carrots, cuts into chunks
1 parsnip, cut into chunks
1 courgette, thickly sliced
4 garlic cloves, thickly sliced
1 red bell pepper, de-seeded
and cut into chunks
2 tbsp olive oil
2 tbsp soy sauce
Ground black pepper
Fresh or dried mixed herbs

Serves 4

Method

1. Preheat oven to 180°C (350°F).
2. Arrange cut vegetables onto a large baking tray and drizzle with olive oil and soy sauce. Mix well. Add herbs and season with pepper.
3. Roast vegetables for 20 minutes. Remove from oven and turn vegetables over.
4. Bake for an additional 10 minutes, or until vegetables are tender and slightly browned.

Try me out

Tip: To make tasty nutritious chips, heat oven to 200°C (400°F). In a shallow roasting tin, toss sweet potato (cut into chips) with olive or coconut oil, soy sauce and seasoning. Bake for 30–40 minutes until crisp.

WAY 38

Turn to turmeric for curcumin cure

When Marco Polo discovered turmeric on his travels through China in the 13th century, he declared it 'a vegetable which has all the properties of true saffron, as well as the smell, the colour, and yet is not really saffron' (59).

Turmeric has been used extensively in medicinal preparations or as a food-colouring agent since 600 BC. Nowadays, it is no longer regarded as a cheaper version of saffron but an exotic spice and colouring agent with outstanding health benefits.

The turmeric plant grows in tropical conditions, is closely related to ginger and has a similar-shaped, brilliant orange-coloured root. Once the root has been dried and ground, it becomes deep yellow in colour, with a distinctive earthy flavour. Curry just wouldn't look or taste the same without it.

In Ancient China and India, turmeric was revered as an anti-inflammatory medicine to treat infections, digestive and respiratory problems, as well as many other conditions. The yellow pigment, curcumin, is the biologically most active compound in turmeric. A potent anti-inflammatory, curcumin may provide similar reductions in pain and swelling in arthritic conditions as prescription drugs, but without the side-effects (60). There is great interest in curcumin as a promising agent in other conditions which also have an inflammatory component, such as heart disease, obesity and Type 2 diabetes. A multitude of studies also suggest anti-oxidant, antiviral and antimicrobial activities. Interestingly, curcumin is substantially more bioavailable when consumed with piperine, a compound derived from black pepper (61). In modern India, the popularity of turmeric is such that it is used in almost all vegetable and meat dishes. India also has one of the lowest rates of Alzheimer's Disease. Researchers are now suggesting that curcumin may be involved in reducing oxidative damage, inflammation and the accumulation of plaque deposits in the brain.

In test tube and animal studies, curcumin also appears effective in cancer prevention. Curcumin affects cellular signalling pathways, including those that mediate proliferation, invasion and metastasis. Scientists have demonstrated that curcumin suppresses specific proteins which promote abnormal inflammatory responses, implying the curry compound may inhibit the progression of cancer. However, research is still preliminary and human studies are needed to confirm curcumin's potential in cancer prevention or treatment.

Turmeric is available as a spice or in tablets or capsules for therapeutic use. If pregnant, suffering from gallstones or other disorders of the bile duct, avoid consuming large amounts. When using turmeric in cooking, try to find an organically grown, non-irradiated version and store in a cool, dark and dry place. Turmeric was used to preserve food well before man-made preservatives were introduced. Add it to egg salad, brown rice, curries, fish and chicken dishes, lentils and salad dressings.

SEE ALSO
- **WAY 16: Butter is better** (page 54)
- **WAY 22: Garlic is 'as good as ten mothers'** (page 66)

Red Lentils with Turmeric, Garlic and Onions

Turmeric provides flavour and its golden colour to this nourishing lentil stew.

Ingredients

2 cups uncooked red lentils, rinsed

4 cups water

$\frac{1}{2}$ tsp ground turmeric

1–2 tsp ghee

1 large red onion, chopped

4 cloves garlic, minced

6 cups cooked brown basmati rice

Sea salt and freshly ground black
pepper to taste

Serves 6

Method

1 Bring lentils, turmeric and water to a boil
   in a pot. Reduce heat and simmer until
   lentils are very soft and pulpy, around
   25 minutes, then set aside.

2 Heat ghee in a large pan over medium
   heat. Add onions and garlic and cook
   until soft, taking care not to burn them.

3 Add onion mixture to lentils and stir well.
   Season with salt and
   black pepper. Serve
   hot, with basmati rice
   on the side.

Tip: The main phytonutrient in black pepper (piperine) can significantly increase
the body's uptake of curcumin, so remember to add some freshly ground black pepper
to dishes containing turmeric.

RECIPE VARIATIONS AND SUBSTITUTIONS

RECIPE VARIATIONS
AND SUBSTITUTIONS

RECIPE VARIATIONS AND SUBSTITUTIONS

RECIPE VARIATIONS
AND SUBSTITUTIONS

1 2 3 4 5 6 7 8
9 10 11 12 13 14
15 16 17 18 19
20 21 22 23 24
25 26 27 28 29
30 31 32 33 34
35 36 37 38 **39**
40 41 42 43 44
45 46 47 48 49

Chapter 3

SNACKS AND DESSERTS

Healthy eating is all about enjoying, not depriving yourself. Prepare fresh raw juices to energise you and throw together a tasty home-made trail mix, roasted seeds or flapjacks to take with you when out and about. Indulge in delectable desserts knowing that these are actually good for you. Even chocolate is 'allowed' if it is the antioxidant-rich variety containing 70% cacao or more. Delicious, protein-packed treats and fuss-free desserts can be low in sugar, yet nutrient-dense and satisfying all at the same time.

WAY 39

Avocado, the fruit of paradise

'The avocado is a food without rival among the fruits, the veritable fruit of paradise.'

So David Fairchild (1869–1954), the famous American botanist and plant explorer is widely quoted as saying. The pear-shaped fruit, originally from Central America, has been consumed for more than 5,000 years. Its name was derived from the Aztec 'ahuacatl' (meaning 'testicle'). Widely cultivated around the world, the plant has been used for a number of medicinal purposes including the treatment of dysentery, and also topically for wound healing and hair growth. One of the most popular varieties is the dark-skinned Hass, due to its flavour, availability and ripening characteristics.

The avocado is known as a 'whole food'. It has the highest protein content among any fruit and contains all essential amino acids, although not in the same density as meat or eggs (62). Avocados are an excellent source of fibre, folate, vitamins E, C, B5, B6 and the minerals iron, copper and magnesium. Exceptionally rich in potassium, yet low in sodium, regular consumption of avocados may aid in the regulation of blood pressure and protect against circulatory diseases.

Avocados contain plant compounds beneficial for human health such as lutein, a deep yellow plant pigment with anti-oxidant properties. Lutein is a member of the carotenoid family (such as beta- and alpha-carotene, lycopene, zeaxanthin) and is thought to benefit eye health as it protects against the damaging effects of strong light. Our ability to absorb the important fat-soluble carotenoids improves when eating avocados as they contain the fatty acids required for easier absorption.

Many people avoid eating avocados precisely because they are high in fat. However, the unsaturated and monounsaturated avocado oils have known health benefits. Eaten in moderation, these beneficial oils provide a feeling of satiety and reduce cravings and the tendency to overeat. The much-maligned avocado is in fact a useful 'aid' for controlling blood sugar fluctuations and weight.

Diets high in monounsaturated fatty acids have another hidden bonus. They improve blood lipids by reducing total blood cholesterol, and by increasing the ratio of high-density lipoprotein (HDL) to the more damaging low-density lipoprotein (LDL) (63). Lipoproteins transport cholesterol around the body. The so-called 'bad' LDLs carry cholesterol from the liver to the cells and may, in excess, cause a harmful build-up of cholesterol. The 'good' HDLs take cholesterol from the cells back to the liver to be excreted.

The luscious, creamy avocado lends itself perfectly to a simple breakfast or snack and is super nutritious – all you need is a spoon to scoop out the tasty flesh. Perfect during pregnancy due to its high folate levels, avocados are also useful during the weaning process as infants can digest them easily. Anyone with a latex allergy should be cautious as they may react to some foods, including avocado.

SEE ALSO
● **WAY 25: Lemon Aid** (page 72)

Avocado Dip (Guacamole)

Quick, simple and tasty version of the classic recipe.
A ripe avocado yields slightly to gentle pressure.

Ingredients

2 ripe avocados
1–2 tbsp lime or lemon juice
Pinch of sea salt
Optional garnishes: red
onion, minced garlic,
chopped parsley
or coriander

Serves 2–4

Method

1. Peel avocados, place in bowl and sprinkle with lemon juice and salt.
2. Mash avocados with a fork until spreadable but still lumpy.
3. Make just before serving as the dip will discolour rapidly. Serve with raw vegetables cut into bite-sized strips.

Tip: To prevent discolouration rub avocado slices with lemon or lime juice. For a simple, tasty and energy-boosting snack on the go, cut the avocado lengthwise working around the pit, release, discard the pit, then put the halves back together, wrap and add to your lunchbox.

WAY 40

Beetroot, can you beat it?

Love it or hate it, beetroot is rarely treated with indifference. For some, the taste of this root vegetable is as overpowering as its vibrant red-violet colour. Others enjoy its extraordinary sweet, earthy taste and its versatility.

Juiced, shredded, pickled, baked or steamed – beetroot is a wonderful accompaniment to most dishes. Or simply do as the Eastern Europeans and create a delicious beetroot soup, also known as borscht.

Beets are packed with nutrients. They contain potassium, magnesium, folic acid, iron, zinc, calcium, phosphorus, sodium, niacin, biotin, vitamin B6 and fibre. Water-soluble pigments called betacyanins are responsible for providing beetroot with its dark red, crimson or purple colouring. Betacyanins are plant compounds currently being studied for their anti-oxidant and anti-inflammatory properties. Researchers at Oxford Brookes University have discovered that concentrated beetroot juice has a unique anti-oxidant profile, and that it appears to be more bioavailable than many other vegetable juices (64).

Beetroot is also high in dietary nitrate. Nitrates in vegetables such as beetroot and spinach produce a naturally occurring gas called nitric oxide in the blood which can help to open blood vessels and improve blood flow and oxygen delivery throughout the body. Although we continuously make our own nitric oxide, production can be increased by the consumption of natural dietary nitrates. In medicine, nitrate-containing medicines are used as vasodilators to relax and widen the blood vessels, allowing more blood and oxygen to flow to the heart, and these are used to treat the chest pain associated with angina.

According to recent research from Reading University, consuming beetroot juice or beetroot-enriched bread can significantly lower blood pressure (65). Other UK based research suggests that in addition to its cardio-protective effects, beetroot juice improves blood flow to the brain and may provide dietary support in the fight against cognitive decline and dementia. Due to its effect of generating more oxygen in the blood, there are also reports that beetroot juice improves stamina and endurance during exercise and aids muscle recovery.

Traditionally, beetroot has been regarded as an effective gallbladder cleanser responsible for stimulating bile flow, and has commonly been used to treat digestive conditions. When cooking or steaming beets, wash rather than peel them to prevent the colour from leeching out and staining your kitchen equipment. Used for centuries as a dye for food and clothes, the colour of beetroot is so potent that after eating it, your urine may be infused with pink. There is no need for alarm, this is completely normal.

SEE ALSO
- **WAY 3: Apples are as good they say, better in fact** (page 22)
- **WAY 7: Fire up your digestion with ginger** (page 30)
- **WAY 18: Celery, a dose of Hippocrates's medicine** (page 58)

Beetroot, Carrot and Orange Juice

Beetroot juice has a wonderful sweet, earthy taste and is incredibly energising.

Ingredients

2 beets, peeled

1 carrot, peeled

1 orange, freshly squeezed

1 apple, chopped

1 stick of celery, chopped

1cm piece fresh ginger,
chopped or sliced (optional)

Serves 2

Method

1. Scrub the vegetables using a stiff vegetable brush.
2. Top and tail the beetroot and carrots if organic, otherwise peel.
3. Chop the vegetables and apple into pieces to fit your juicer.
4. Juice the vegetables and apple, then add the orange juice and serve immediately. Beetroot juice is very concentrated, so needs to be diluted with water.

Try me out

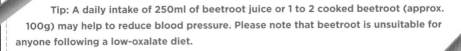

Tip: A daily intake of 250ml of beetroot juice or 1 to 2 cooked beetroot (approx. 100g) may help to reduce blood pressure. Please note that beetroot is unsuitable for anyone following a low-oxalate diet.

WAY 41 Chocolate, you are simply divine

If God had wanted women to be perfect, he would not have invented chocolate.

Creating a food as sumptuously soothing, as voluptuously velvety as chocolate was a rotten trick to play, especially on nutritionists who are supposed to abstain at all times. Apart from Christmas, Valentine's Day, Easter, Mother's Day, Birthdays, Unbirthdays and... no doubt we can think of something.

There is no end to our wickedness where chocolate is concerned. We shamelessly turn out our partners' pockets, not for signs of infidelity but the tag-end of an antique chocolate bar. And are prone to making rash promises if only he will go out to replenish our dwindling supplies at all hours and in all weathers. Real heroes always comply, just like the chap in the famous Milk Tray ad, for there is no greater fury to behold than a woman deprived of her favourite chocolate.

But is it good for us? Chocolate contains the stimulants caffeine and theobromine and large amounts of sugar, so it is used by many people as an instant lift when energy levels are low. The cocoa bean contains several important minerals including magnesium, copper, zinc and iron. Women suffering from PMS may be low in magnesium and find they are less able to control their cravings for chocolate at that time. It also contains phenylethylamine, a natural mood enhancer which stimulates the brain's pleasure and reward centres.

The Aztec Emperor Montezuma (1480–1520) was renowned for using chocolate as an aphrodisiac by drinking a cup whenever he visited his wives. Known as 'Food of the Gods', cacao beans were revered by the Aztecs and Mayans so highly they were used as a form of currency. Unlike the modern heat-treated, over-processed and sugar-laden versions, raw chocolate has impressive medicinal properties and was used for centuries in Central and South America in healing rituals. Luckily, authentic raw organic chocolate can now be found in health stores or ordered online.

Dried at low temperatures, raw cacao is a highly nutritious, slightly bitter powder that can be formed into bars, nibs, smoothies and delicious deserts, or used as a substitute for coffee. Cacao flavonols promote a healthy cardiovascular system by improving blood flow, elasticity of blood vessels and insulin resistance (66). Further studies also report benefits for brain and gut health.

Montezuma is quoted as saying that chocolate is 'the divine drink, which builds up resistance and fights fatigue. A cup of this precious drink permits a man to walk for a whole day without food'. Look for products containing a minimum of 70% or more cocoa solids. Whenever cocoa is listed after sugar and fat, however, it really is best avoided.

SEE ALSO
- **WAY 4: Berry healthy for you** (page 24)
- **WAY 47: Seeds: all good things come in small packages** (page 122)

Raw Chocolate Trail Mix

This is a fabulous and energising snack to enjoy when in need of a boost.
Please note that cocoa nibs contain caffeine, and should be consumed in moderation.

Ingredients
$^1/_2$ cup raw cocoa nibs
1 cup sunflower seeds
1 cup pumpkin seeds
1 cup goji berries
$^1/_2$ cup dried cranberries
$^1/_2$ cup dried mulberries or sultanas

Makes approximately 10–12 servings

Method
Mix all the ingredients together (commonly found separately in healthfood stores) and store in a large airtight container in the fridge.

Try me out

Tip: If you rely heavily on chocolate for an energy fix instead of more nutritious foods, reduce your intake gradually over several weeks and replace it with alternative snacks or raw chocolate. The best time for a woman to give up chocolate is at the beginning of her menstrual cycle. Within three weeks, she should find her cravings considerably reduced.

42 Cinnamon, add some spice into your life

There is renewed interest in natural remedies such as spices that have been handed down over many generations.

Traditionally spices were used not only to flavour dishes, but to disguise rancid food. Unhygienic food and storage practices, combined with a lack of understanding about germs, made food downright hazardous. Fortunately, some spices exhibit anti-microbial activity, which protected our ancestors from food poisoning.

Cinnamon, one of our most popular baking spices, was discovered on the beautiful island of Sri Lanka (formerly Ceylon). Cut from the dried bark of several species of trees native to South East Asia, it has been used not only as a preservative and natural flavouring, but also in traditional medicines to relieve different ailments.

Recently, there has been scientific interest in cinnamon. The USDA's Nutrient Requirements and Functions Laboratory suggest that $^1/_2$ teaspoon of cinnamon per day improves blood sugar and lipids (67). Cinnamon and its components are thought to boost the efficiency of insulin and may have potential in the prevention and treatment of insulin resistance, metabolic syndrome and Type 2 diabetes (68). In diabetes, glucose carried by the blood cannot reach our cells effectively. Glucose is the body's major source of fuel and we obtain it easily from carbohydrates (sugars and starches) and more slowly from protein and fat. But before we can make use of glucose, it has to be transported around the body and taken up by our cells with the help of insulin. In diabetes, less insulin is produced or cells become resistant to it. Excess glucose starts building up in the blood, leaving body tissues deprived of their main energy source. Treatment, involving diet, exercise and insulin replacement is needed to avoid serious complications.

Numerous studies involving cinnamon in laboratory and animal models have shown beneficial results. Human clinical trials, however, have been less conclusive, possibly because of the dosage and type of cinnamon used, and the variation in the sample population chosen – for example including patients already taking diabetic drugs. The most consistent findings with cinnamon in human trials were improved fasting glucose levels. Impaired fasting glucose levels (a pre-diabetic state) means the body is unable to regulate glucose as efficiently as it should.

Different species of cinnamon differ in chemical composition and properties. Some types contain high levels of the flavouring coumarin which can cause side-effects if consumed in high doses (69). Ceylon cinnamon (C. zeylanicum), however, contains low levels of coumarin and is considered quite safe whilst exhibiting potent anti-oxidant, anti-inflammatory and antibacterial properties and improving blood sugar (70). Diabetics should not significantly alter their diet or discontinue prescribed medication without consulting their physician.

SEE ALSO
- **WAY 45: How to care a fig about your 'five-a-day'** (page 118)

Baked Rice Pudding

Good old-fashioned rice pud is the ultimate comfort food. Enjoy hot or cold.

Ingredients

2 cups (500ml) milk of your choice
(combining soya and coconut
milk works well)

$^1/3$ cup pudding rice

1 tsp ground cinnamon

4–5 pitted dates chopped

Chopped nuts (optional)

1 tbsp butter

Serves 4–6

Method

1. Pre-heat oven to 160°C (325°F).
2. Combine the pudding rice, milk, dates and cinnamon in a greased ovenproof dish. Dot butter over the top.
3. Place in the oven (without a cover) for 30 minutes. Stir well.
4. Bake for a further hour and serve with Fig and Apricot Compote.

Try me out

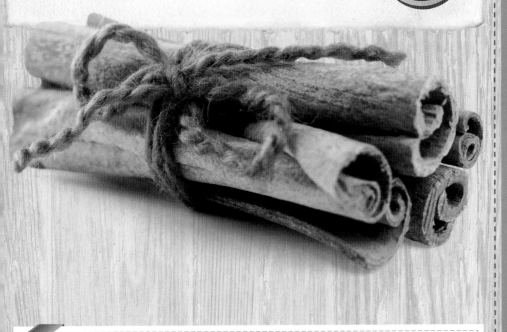

Tip: Store ground cinnamon in a large shaker and sprinkle over herbal tea, coffee, cocoa, pancakes, batter, oats, fruit salad, toast, yoghurt, cottage or ricotta cheese. Soya milk simmered with cinnamon sticks and honey makes a deliciously warming drink.

43

Grapes and the mystery of the French Paradox

We have treasured grapes ever since we discovered that wine could be produced from fermented grape juice.

It has been said that wine can only be as good as the grape from which it is made. But have you ever wondered why it is traditional to buy grapes for people recovering from illness? Grapes are not only tasty and easy to eat, they have useful health benefits.

The skin and seeds of red and purple grapes contain a polyphenol anti-oxidant called resveratrol, a member of the flavonoid family. Flavonoids are plant pigments responsible for the vibrant red, blue and purple colours in fruit and vegetables. Resveratrol is particularly prevalent in grapes, berries, peanuts and some medicinal plants. As it is both water- and fat-soluble, it is highly versatile.

Laboratory and animal studies suggest resveratrol has anti-aging, anti-inflammatory and anti-oxidant properties. Resveratrol may have considerable potential to improve health and prevent chronic disease in humans, too (71). There are, however, still only limited human clinical trials and a lack of data on the bioavailability of resveratrol and the exact dosages required.

The most common and popular dietary source of resveratrol is red wine, which is often cited as a factor in the French Paradox. This is the observation that French people have a low incidence of heart disease, despite drinking alcohol (red wine) and consuming a diet high in saturated fat. The explanation is likely to be multi-factorial and more complex, involving general dietary habits, genes and the environment. Interestingly, resveratrol concentrations in wine vary widely, even within specific grape varieties and growing regions.

In addition to resveratrol, scientists have found another important flavonoid in grapes called quercetin which has natural anti-histamine and anti-inflammatory effects. Grapes are a good source of potassium and have unique cleansing properties. As they contain almost 80% water, they are also a convenient low-calorie snack. Dried grapes, or raisins, are much more concentrated in calories as they contain only 15% water, but they are a valuable source of iron and fibre. Raisins are high in glucose and fructose, providing an instant energy boost for active people, although those with blood sugar problems should avoid eating dried fruit in large quantities.

The anti-oxidant compounds in purple grape juice appear to have a similar effect as those in red wine, assisting the body in neutralising free radicals responsible for cellular damage that may contribute to disease and premature aging. However, grape juice does so without the intoxicating effects of alcohol.

SEE ALSO
- **WAY 11: Pineapple and its super-healing enzyme** (page 38)

Tutti Frutti

Try out other fruit combinations for variety,
including Sharon fruit, plums and melon.

Ingredients

1 red grapefruit, halved

Black grapes

Kiwi fruit, cut into bite-size pieces

Small chunks of pineapple

Toothpicks

*Makes enough to satisfy a large
group if 're-stacked' regularly.*

Method

1. For a healthy and delicious party snack food, cut a large red grapefruit in half and place both halves face down on a large party platter.

2. Thread chunks of pineapple, kiwi and black grapes onto toothpicks and stick these into the grapefruit halves to make a tempting fruity display.

Try me out

Tip: Before popping those luscious grapes into your mouth, make sure you wash them well, as grape skins may be contaminated with moulds and pesticide residues.

WAY 44 — Honey, honey

Raw, unprocessed honey is renowned for its health-giving properties and should be treated with some respect if one considers that an average worker bee only produces 1/12th teaspoon of the golden liquid in its lifetime.

Hardworking bees visit two million flowers to gather enough nectar for merely one pound of honey. Different flowers produce honey with differing tastes and colours and it has been stated that dark honey may provide more anti-oxidants than the lighter varieties.

Honey has been used since ancient times as an antiseptic salve to heal burns and sores. It was one of the most common ingredients in medicines in Ancient Egypt and often used in religious ceremonies. The druids called Britain the 'Isle of Honey' and in Medieval England, honey was so prized that people even paid their taxes with it. A popular brew called mead was made from diluted honey and water and fermented with yeast.

Honey has an established reputation from laboratory studies and clinical trials as an antibacterial agent that has a broad spectrum of activity. Research also indicates that honey displays anti-inflammatory effects and stimulates immune responses. No great surprise then that it has been traditionally used to reduce infection and enhance wound healing in burns, ulcers, and other cutaneous wounds. These effects are believed to be due to a variety of factors, including honey's acidity, hydrogen peroxide content, osmotic effects, nutritional and anti-oxidant ingredients and other, as yet unidentified compounds and mechanisms (72).

Honeys from different geographical areas appear to have differing therapeutic properties. Eating locally produced honey may help to reduce hay fever symptoms. It is also a soothing remedy for sore throats and chesty coughs when mixed with hot water, ginger and lemon juice. Certain varieties show greater promise in treating wounds. The famous Manuka honey from New Zealand is particularly potent and there are anecdotal reports – but no clinical evidence – that it may be helpful in eradicating H pylori, a bacterium responsible for stomach ulcers.

Honey provides both glucose and fructose in a pre-digested form and is sweeter and more rapidly assimilated than refined sugar. Although honey is a healthier option than refined sugar because it contains traces of amino acids, enzymes, minerals and vitamins, it is still a highly concentrated source of sweetness and used by the body in much the same way as sugar. It should be used sparingly if suffering from blood sugar fluctuations and weight issues.

In commercially processed, heat-treated and strained honeys, the natural enzymes and up to 50% of nutrients are lost, along with much of the original flavour and fragrance.

As supermarket honeys are generally a pasteurised and filtered blend of different honeys from different countries, natural cold-pressed local honeys are preferable.

SEE ALSO
- **WAY 2: Almonds, the all-rounder** (page 20)
- **WAY 10: Oat cuisine** (page 36)
- **WAY 16: Butter is better** (page 54)
- **WAY 47: Seeds: all good things come in small packages** (page 122)

Honey Crunch Flapjacks

A very yummy, crunchy version of the favourite cookie bar treat.

Ingredients

225g runny honey
225g butter
350g rolled oats
50g chopped almonds
50g sunflower seeds
75g dates, stoned and chopped

Makes approximately 12 flapjacks

Method

1. Preheat oven to 180°C (350°F) and grease a 30 x 25cm (12in x 9in) square baking tin.

2. Melt the honey with the butter in a large saucepan. Add the rolled oats, almonds, sunflower seeds and chopped dates.

3. Mix well, spoon into the baking tin and spread to about 2cm thick. Smooth the surface with the back of a spoon.

4. Bake for about 20–25 minutes until golden brown but still slightly soft in the middle. Cool in the tin, but cut into squares while still warm.

Tip: Avoid giving honey to infants under the age of one due to the risk of infection by the bacterial spores it may contain. Honey is safe to eat during pregnancy and while breastfeeding, although raw unpasteurised honey should be avoided during this time.

WAY 45
How to care a fig about your 'five-a-day'

We are all aware that eating more fruit and vegetables is good for us as they contain nutrients and plant compounds which protect our cells from the damaging effects of chemicals in our own bodies, as well as in the environment, that can speed up ageing and disease.

Fresh fruit and vegetables also contain valuable amounts of fibre, critically important for nourishing our gut bacteria and helping to eliminate waste and prevent constipation. As an added bonus, eating fruit and vegetables provides us with less inclination or room for unhealthy sugary and fat-laden convenience foods.

Eating five portions, and ideally seven to nine portions a day is easy. For example, one serving equals one piece of medium-sized fruit (apple, banana, orange), or two tablespoons of vegetables (raw or cooked), or one dessert bowlful of salad, or one tablespoon dried fruit, or one glass of fruit juice, or three tablespoons of fresh fruit salad/stewed fruit.

In order to get the most from your fruit and veggies, eat them as soon as possible, wash them thoroughly and don't overcook. Buy organic if you can and, to increase variety, experiment with produce you have never tried before.

Here are some five-a-day tips:

1. Start your day with freshly squeezed fruit juice or a smoothie and add a sliced banana with dried fruit on your cereal or muesli.
2. Keep an apple, bag of carrot sticks or dried apricots in your handbag/briefcase to have as a mid-morning and mid-afternoon snack.
3. Instead of buying a sandwich for lunch, choose a tasty salad with grated or diced vegetables, hummus, tuna or chicken pieces.
4. Add plenty of seasonal vegetables to casseroles or serve two different vegetables with your main meal rather than just one.
5. For dessert, enjoy live yoghurt topped with fresh berries.

One of my favourite fruit is the fig, a member of the mulberry family. Figs contain useful amounts of iron, calcium, potassium and an exceptional amount of fibre. They are commonly used as both food and medicine in the Middle East, and many different varieties exist. The fruits may be eaten raw, dried or stewed, made into jams or wine, and included as a natural sweetener for beverages, porridge and puddings.

Mrs Beeton, of legendary cookbook fame, can be credited for using figs as the main ingredient in her Christmas puddings. Traditionally figs were used as an effective laxative to prevent chronic constipation, relieve catarrh and to soothe inflamed mucous membranes in the throat and chest. Ancient Greek Olympians consumed figs to increase their speed and strength, and prized them so highly they were crowned with fig wreaths.

SEE ALSO
- **WAY 42: Cinnamon, add some spice into your life** (page 112)

Fig and Apricot Compote

A compote of dried fruits is a simple but delicious dessert. Soak a handful of dried figs and apricots overnight, then simmer gently with cinnamon until soft. Serve warm with baked rice pudding or cold with live yoghurt.

Tip: Dried figs and other dried fruit are often treated with preservatives called sulphites which may cause adverse reactions in those with allergies and asthma. Check labels and buy organic varieties.

WAY 46 Liquid veggies, fresh and raw

Staying away from junk food isn't easy. Fast food outlets specialise in catering for eyes, nose and taste buds rather than well-being. Therein lies the fastest route to your wallet.

My advice is to scrutinise processed foods – don't get taken in by the wholesome images on the packaging. Check labels carefully to see whether the food actually contains the suggested nutritious items or is made mostly from artificial ingredients and fillers. Some manufacturers replace E-numbers with the full chemical name of the food additive in order to make their product appear more wholesome than it really is.

Best of all, forsake 'junk' and treat yourself to a big, green leafy salad every day. Here's how: make a base of organic green salad leaves and top with whatever fresh vegetables are to hand, for example grated carrots, courgettes, chopped tomatoes, spring onions, olives, avocado, red or yellow peppers. Make it as colourful as a rainbow. Then add some protein such as sliced egg, hummus, pieces of fish or chicken and finally, splash on some dressing. Those who regularly eat salads and raw vegetables have higher levels of key nutrients promoting health and reducing the risk of obesity, heart disease and other chronic degenerative illnesses.

If you don't enjoy eating salads or vegetables, you can drink them. Instead of your usual glass of plain orange, try juicing an apple with a few chunks of raw carrot and beetroot. Vegetable juicing offers an efficient method of extracting sugars, starches, proteins and enzymes in a concentrated form that is easy to consume and absorb. For your efforts you receive an instant energy and immune booster which looks glorious and tastes delicious. Whizz up different combinations of ingredients and create your own unique blends – fresh, additive-free and unpasteurised.

Apple and carrot are good bases and can be mixed with all other fruit and vegetables. Try celery, spinach, pepper, watercress, sweet potato, cucumber, tomato or parsnip. Avoid large quantities of fruit or carrot juices, however, as they upset blood sugar levels and contribute to weight gain. Always dilute your juices with water as they are so highly concentrated.

Support local organic farms as non-organic fruit, salad and vegetables may be contaminated with pesticide residues. A report has found that the use of pesticides rose by 6.5% between 2005 and 2010 (73). We are assured that minute levels of pesticides present no health risk to consumers, but only a small selection of produce are tested at any one time. There is also concern about long-term low doses and the cumulative effects of all residues. Play safe by scrubbing all fresh produce thoroughly under running water to remove not only traces of chemicals but any dirt and bacteria. Discard outer leaves of leafy vegetables and eat a variety of foods from different sources to reduce exposure to any single pesticide.

Green Energy Juice No 1

Start your day off with one of these hydrating and super nutritious green juices.

Ingredients
2 cups of water
3 carrots, peeled
2 stalks celery, washed
1 turnip, peeled
A couple of handfuls of spinach, washed
A handful of parsley

Serves 2

Method
Run all the ingredients through the juice extractor and dilute with water, depending on how strong you like your veggie juices.

Green Energy Juice No 2

Ingredients
2 cups of water
$1/2$ chopped cucumber
1 stick celery
$1/4$ of a chopped fennel bulb
$1/2$ avocado
1 tbsp parsley
1 clove garlic (optional)
Juice of $1/2$ lemon
Pinch of seasalt or dash of tamari soy sauce
A couple of handfuls of spinach leaves

Serves 2-3

Method
Combine all the ingredients in a blender and whizz until smooth. Add more water if required.

(Recipe adapted from a version by Nadia Brydon)

Tip: Lettuce may have sedative effects. Wild lettuce was used as a traditional herbal remedy to induce sleep and calm restlessness and anxiety. To improve sleep, juice some fresh organic lettuce to make up a small cup and flavour with a few drops of lemon juice.

47

Seeds: all good things come in small packages

Treat yourself to one of nature's ultimate convenience foods – so easy to prepare and display. They may be small, but sunflower, pumpkin and hemp seeds are packed with mighty nutritional gems.

High in fibre, they contain vitamins, minerals and plant protein, as well as those all-important essential fatty acids required for growth, development and repair. Best eaten raw, tossed into salads, stir-fries or any grain and vegetable dish for an added 'crunch' factor.

Pumpkins produce one of the tastiest and most nutritious of all seeds – about a cupful of seeds each. These are an excellent source of fibre as well as the minerals zinc, magnesium, potassium and iron. Pumpkin seeds have many reputed health benefits and were traditionally used as an intestinal anti-parasitic. Men, in particular, should consider eating a handful of these seeds daily as researchers have found the essential oils and plant sterols in pumpkin seeds may prove beneficial in the management of benign prostatic hyperplasia or 'enlarged prostate' (74). Human clinical trials, however, are required to substantiate this.

Sunflower seeds, another popular and nutritious snack, are a rich source of vitamin E, vitamin B6 and the minerals magnesium, iron, zinc and selenium. Native Americans ate sunflower seeds raw or ground them to make breads and cakes. They were also used in medical ointments. Sunflower seeds are high in omega-6 fatty acids, an essential fat the body cannot produce on its own, and they contain plant sterols which may help to modify blood cholesterol levels.

Of all the seeds, hemp seeds are the most perfectly balanced, containing essential nutrients and complete protein in an easily digestible form. Unlike other seeds, hemp seeds also contain both omega-3 and omega-6 fatty acids in the right proportions for long-term use, resulting in improved cell membrane function and decreased inflammatory processes in the body.

Those with skin problems should take particular note of hempseed oil's mild-tasting, greenish oil following the findings of Finnish researchers who saw a reduction in dryness, itching and an overall improvement in the symptoms of eczema after daily consumption (75). Adults can take 1–2 tablespoons of hempseed oil (children 1–2 teaspoons) daily in order to maintain a balanced source of essential fatty acids. Use hempseed oil as a salad dressing or mix with spreads, juices or smoothies.

All seeds are delicious as snacks for children in between meals – lightly toasting them brings out their flavour. Another way to use them is to grind your seeds in a clean coffee grinder and sprinkle the resulting seed meal over your breakfast muesli or yoghurt.

SEE ALSO
• **WAY 48: The wonderful world of flax** (page 124)

Roasted Mixed Seeds

Roasted seeds are an invaluable addition to your salads and stir-fries.
They also make wonderful savoury snacks.

Ingredients

$1/2$ cup sunflower seeds

$1/2$ cup pumpkin seeds

2 tsp Tamari soy sauce
or a sprinkling
of sea salt

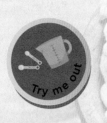

Try me out

Method

1. Mix seeds with soy sauce and arrange in thin layer on a baking tray.
2. Bake at a low temperature at 160°C (325°F) in the oven for approximately 10–15 minutes until lightly browned. Watch carefully as the seeds brown and burn easily. Cool and store in an airtight container in the fridge.

Tip: Seeds and their cold-pressed oils should be stored in airtight containers in the fridge and not heated as the essential fats are very delicate and easily damaged by exposure to light, heat and air.

WAY 48 The wonderful world of flax

The Latin name for flaxseed is Linum usitatissimum and means 'most useful'. Flax has been used as food and textile fibre for over 5000 years and remains an important functional food. It has favourable effects on immunity, hormones and digestion, and significant potential in disease prevention (76).

Before the Second World War, the 'multitalented' flax was fairly common in the European diet. Now it is once again increasing in popularity as the richest vegetarian source of omega-3 essential fatty acids (EFAs). Fatty acids are components of our cell membranes, affecting the flexibility and permeability of all body cells. They prevent loss of moisture from our skin and mucous membranes, are required for the structure and function of the brain and are mediators in controlling blood pressure, immunity and many other physiological activities. The body cannot manufacture its own EFAs, so we are entirely dependent on dietary sources.

For optimal health, we need to obtain enough of two groups of EFAs: omega-6 and omega-3 in the right proportions. The omega-6s are found in nuts, seeds and most vegetable oils. The richest source of omega-3s comes from cold-water fish, then flaxseed, and there are smaller amounts in walnuts, wheat germ and soya oils. Researchers are concerned that our modern diet is particularly lacking in the omega-3 oils. For vegetarians and those worried about polluted or farmed fish, flax is a welcome alternative. There is however, considerable individual variation in our ability to readily convert the simpler form of omega-3 from flaxseeds (ALA) into the required EPA and DHA (found in fish and seafood).

The tiny flaxseeds are golden or brown in colour with a pleasant, nutty flavour. Packed with fibre and soothing mucilage which coat the digestive tract, they ease the passage of stools and help to prevent constipation. Simply grind one tablespoon of flaxseeds in a coffee grinder and sprinkle over cereal. Or add flaxseeds to a glass of water, leave to soak overnight, and add to your porridge. Always drink plenty of water when adding flaxseed to your diet.

The flaxseed hull is a concentrated source of lignans, a type of phytoestrogen. Lignans are converted by our intestinal bacteria into hormone-like substances that appear to have anti-carcinogenic effects. The phytoestrogenic and anti-oxidant properties of lignans may also ease menopausal symptoms and there is evidence they may protect against cardiovascular disease, osteoporosis and diabetes.

Whole flaxseeds can stay fresh for up to a year if stored correctly but will go rancid more quickly once ground up. Add a few flaxseeds to your bowl of soup, casseroles, meatloaf or meatballs. Flaxseed oil (available in capsule or liquid form) should be refrigerated and never heated as essential oils are volatile and spoil quickly when exposed to heat, light or oxygen. Discard the oil if it tastes bitter or rancid. Use a tablespoon of flaxseed oil a day instead of salad dressings, or mix it into juice and yoghurt.

SEE ALSO

- **WAY 41: Chocolate, you are simply divine** (page 110)
- **WAY 42: Cinnamon, add some spice into your life** (page 112)
- **WAY 49: Versatile bananas for high energy** (page 126)

Fruit and Flaxseed Dessert

A mouth-watering dessert that can also be enjoyed for breakfast.

Ingredients

A handful of frozen blueberries or
1 apple peeled and cut into chunks
1 banana
Juice of one orange
3 tbsp ground flaxseed
6 soaked almonds (soak for 3 hours
or overnight)
1–2 tbsp milk or milk alternative
$1/2$ tsp cinnamon
Raw chocolate nibs

Serves 2

Method

1. Place all ingredients in a food processor except the chocolate nibs and puree until smooth.
2. Spoon into bowls, sprinkle with raw chocolate nibs and enjoy.

Instead of the nibs you can also use plain 70% dark chocolate and shave off curls using a cheese slicer or potato peeler.

Try me out

Tip: 15g ground flaxseed steeped in 45ml water for two minutes can be used as a substitute for one egg. Flaxseed is gluten-free and when ground, is a healthy replacement for some of the flour in bread, muffin, biscuit and pancake recipes.

WAY 49
Versatile bananas for high energy

For taste and versatility, you can't beat a banana.

Bananas are a good source of magnesium, vitamins C and B6 and an excellent source of potassium, which offsets sodium and helps to regulate blood pressure. They are high in easily digestible carbohydrates and are popular with athletes as natural high-energy snacks. The fibre in ripe bananas promotes good digestion and encourages the production of butyric acid, a substance that protects our delicate internal gut membranes.

Unripe (green) bananas contain resistant starch which is either not digested or only partially digested until it reaches the large intestine where it undergoes bacterial fermentation. It is low glycaemic index (GI) as it is more slowly digested. Resistant starch is currently being investigated for its potential health benefits in blood sugar regulation and weight control (77).

Overripe bananas on the other hand have a high glycaemic response. This means that blood sugar levels rise, demanding the use of more insulin. The glycaemic index is a way of measuring how quickly a carbohydrate enters the bloodstream and how high it raises blood glucose. Eating a banana that has not fully ripened produces a lower glycaemic response and is therefore more suitable for those who find it hard to control their blood sugar levels. The only caveat is that unripe bananas are more difficult to digest.

Bananas also have a natural antacid effect and are thought to reduce the risk of ulcers by creating a barrier between the acid and stomach lining. In India, some doctors treat ulcers with the powder made from members of the banana family called plantains. Plantains (and green bananas) are best cooked before eating.

Choose organic bananas as the skin is highly porous and may absorb pesticides, and avoid storing unripe bananas in the fridge because the cold interferes with the ripening process. Once bananas are completely ripe with yellow skin and tiny brown flecks, they can be refrigerated for up to two weeks wrapped in newspaper, although the skin will turn brown.

Bananas can improve your sense of well-being as they contain the amino acid tryptophan required to produce serotonin, a brain chemical that regulates your mood and helps you sleep. Ideal fast food on the go, a banana is beautifully wrapped in 'legitimate' packaging. No waste here – you can use the skin for a variety of purposes. An insect bite can be relieved by rubbing the affected area with the inside of a banana skin. If you want to remove a wart, cut a small piece of banana skin and place it on the wart, yellow side out. Cover and keep it in place with a plaster, exchanging it for a new bit of banana skin every day. Banana skin can even be used to wipe down the leaves of houseplants to add gloss, or cut into small pieces for plant food.

SEE ALSO
- **WAY 41: Chocolate, you are simply divine** (page 110)

Chocolate Banana Wrap

Enjoy as an occasional 'decadent' treat – it is completely delicious!

Ingredients

2 bananas in their skin

85g dark chocolate (70%)
broken into pieces

2 scoops vanilla ice
cream (optional)

Serves 2

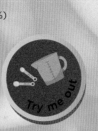

Method

1. Make a slit down the length of the bananas and break the chocolate into pieces, placing some inside each banana skin.

2. Bake the bananas in their skins on a barbecue or in a 200°C (400°F) hot oven for 15–20 minutes until blackened all over. Scoop out and serve with vanilla ice cream.

Tip: Blend a banana, a handful of frozen blueberries and live yoghurt to make a delicious shake. If you have a surplus of ripe bananas, simply peel and cut into chunks, then store in a plastic bag in the freezer. Use the frozen banana chunks for ice-cold smoothies.

RECIPE VARIATIONS
AND SUBSTITUTIONS

RECIPE VARIATIONS
AND SUBSTITUTIONS

RECIPE VARIATIONS
AND SUBSTITUTIONS

RECIPE VARIATIONS
AND SUBSTITUTIONS

RECIPE VARIATIONS
AND SUBSTITUTIONS

RECIPE VARIATIONS
AND SUBSTITUTIONS

GLOSSARY

Amino acids
The basic chemical units or 'building blocks' that make up proteins. They are also synthesized in the body and found in food.

Anthocyanins
Water-soluble plant pigments responsible for giving red, dark blue and purple fruits and vegetables their colour. According to research, these compounds have considerable anti-oxidant and anti-inflammatory effects.

Antioxidant
Any substance that reduces or prevents oxidative damage to cells such as that caused by sunlight or environmental pollutants. The body produces some antioxidants, others are obtained from food.

Antimicrobial
A substance that kills or inhibits the growth of microorganisms such as bacteria, fungi or protozoans.

Avenanthramides
Polyphenol compounds found exclusively in oats. Known to have antioxidant effects and may also inhibit the pro-inflammatory processes associated with atherosclerotic disease.

Beta-carotene
Beta-carotene is a plant pigment from the carotenoid family that the body can convert into vitamin A. Dark green and orange–yellow vegetables are good sources of beta-carotene.

Beta-glucan
Beta-glucan is a type of soluble fibre found in cereal grains. Oats and barley are known to be particularly rich sources. Beta-glucan has immune-stimulating properties and an important role in blood sugar and cholesterol management.

Bifidobacteria
A form of 'friendly' bacteria that reside in the lower part of the digestive system.

Biotin
A water-soluble B-complex vitamin found in egg yolk, liver and yeast. It is required for the metabolism of protein, fats and carbohydrates.

Bromelain
A natural proteolytic enzyme (an enzyme that digests proteins) found in the stem and fruit of the pineapple.

Carotenoids
Yellow, orange and red pigments with antioxidant effects found in many fruit and vegetables.

Choline
An essential nutrient similar to a B vitamin. It is used in many chemical reactions in the body and is particularly important for the integrity of cell membranes.

Circadian rhythm
The body's 24-hour cycle of sleep and wakefulness. It is related to light exposure and shifts in hormone levels.

Collagen
A protein that helps to form bones, cartilage, skin, joints and other tissues in the body.

Enzyme inhibitors
Molecules which bind to enzymes and decrease or block their activity.

Enzymes
Proteins that speed up chemical reactions in the body. Digestive enzymes, for example, help us to break down food.

Fibre
An essential component of our diet from plant-based foods that helps the bowel to pass food, expel waste and control blood sugar. There are two types of fibre: insoluble and soluble.

Flavonoids/flavonols
A large group of plant compounds beneficial to human health. Flavanols are a distinct group of compounds within the flavonoid family and the predominant flavonoids in tea, red wine and cocoa.

Folic acid/folate
One of the B vitamins. Folate is naturally occurring and present in many foods, especially dark green vegetables. Folic acid is synthetically derived in a laboratory.

Glycaemic Index (GI)
Indicator of the ability of different types of foods that contain carbohydrate to raise blood glucose levels within two hours. Carbohydrate-containing foods that break down most quickly during digestion have the highest glycaemic index.

Glycaemic control
A medical term referring to the typical levels of blood sugar (glucose). For diabetics, glycaemic control is a primary goal.

Gingerol
One of the active constituents of fresh ginger.

High-density lipoprotein (HDL)
Also known as 'good' cholesterol and positively associated with a decreased risk of coronary heart disease.

Hyperin
A medicinally active compound found in various plants.

Iodine
A mineral necessary for normal cell metabolism. Required by the thyroid gland in the synthesis and secretion of hormones. Food sources: sea fish, shellfish, seaweed, eggs, dairy, iodized salt.

Iron
Iron is an important mineral required for the production of haemoglobin, the component of red blood cells that transports oxygen around the body. It is also needed to produce myoglobin, which carries oxygen to our muscles. Iron deficiency is one of the most common nutritional deficiencies.

Kefir
A cultured milk drink popular in the Middle East and Eastern Europe, consisting of a complex mixture of lactic acid bacteria and 'friendly' yeasts.

Lactic acid

An organic acid produced by the body during the breakdown of glucose when oxygen is in short supply. Also produced by bacteria during fermentation of foods such as dairy products and sauerkraut.

Lactobacilli

Bacteria found mainly in the mouth, intestinal tract and vagina. Lactobacilli also live in fermenting products like live yoghurt or kefir.

Low-density lipoprotein (LDL)

One of two types of lipoproteins (particles made of proteins and lipids) in the blood that transport cholesterol. Also known as 'bad' cholesterol.

L-Theanine

An amino acid present in tea (Camellia sinensis) , particularly green tea, with known neurological properties.

Lutein

A yellow carotenoid pigment found in plants, animal fats and egg yolk. Thought to be beneficial to eye health.

Lycopene

A red carotenoid pigment present in tomatoes and many berries and fruits. May be beneficial for the health of the prostate.

Magnesium

The fourth most abundant mineral in the body and essential to good health. Green vegetables, legumes, nuts and whole grains are all good sources of magnesium.

Manganese

An essential trace mineral found mostly in whole grains, green leafy vegetables, dried fruits and nuts.

Melatonin

A hormone secreted by the pineal gland (especially in response to darkness) which has been linked to the regulation of circadian rhythms.

Mineral

An inorganic substance, such as calcium, that plays an essential role in the human body.

Monounsaturated fat

A 'good' dietary fat found in foods such as nuts, olive oil, canola oil, and grape seed oil. Can help to lower blood cholesterol if used in place of saturated fats.

Omega-3 (fatty acids)

A class of essential fatty acids found primarily in fish oils, especially from salmon and other cold-water fish. EPA (eicosapentaenoic acid) and DHA (docosahexaenoic acid) are the two principle omega-3 fatty acids.

Omega-6 (fatty acids)

A class of essential fatty acids found in seeds and nuts, and the oils extracted from them. GLA (Gamma-linolenic acid) is a principle omega-6 fatty acid found primarily in hemp, borage and evening primrose oil.

Phenolic compounds

Chemical compounds that possess strong antiseptic and antibacterial properties. Fruits, vegetables and beverages (wine) are the major sources of phenolic compounds in the human diet. Can be manufactured and used in disinfectants, preservatives, dyes, pesticides and medical and industrial chemicals.

Phosphorus
An essential element in the diet and a major component of bone, but also found in blood, muscles, nerves and teeth.

Phytochemicals (phytonutrients)
A large group of compounds produced by plants to protect them from toxins and environmental pollutants. Although not considered essential, they may help to protect against degenerative diseases.

Pineal gland
A tiny gland located in the middle of the brain that produces melatonin.

Plant sterols
Steroid compounds similar to cholesterol which occur in plants, that may help to reduce cholesterol levels.

Polyphenols
A group of chemical substances with antioxidant and anti-inflammatory properties found in berries, walnuts, olives, tea leaves, grapes and many other plants.

Polyunsaturated fat
A highly unsaturated fat that is liquid at room temperature. Found mostly in nuts, seeds, fish, algae and leafy greens.

Potassium
An electrolyte and mineral that plays a major role in maintaining fluid and acid–base balance and assists in regulating neuromuscular activity.

Prebiotics
Prebiotics are specialized plant fibres that provide a food source for the 'friendly' bacteria in our intestines and encourage their growth.

Probiotics
Cultures of live microorganisms that can be ingested to improve the balance of natural microflora in the digestive tract.

Proteins
One or more chains of amino acids. They are required for the structure, function and regulation of the body's cells, tissues and organs. Each protein has unique functions.

Proteolytic enzymes
A group of enzymes that break up the long chainlike molecules of proteins into shorter fragments (peptides) and eventually into their components, amino acids.

Quercetin
A plant–derived flavonoid with anti-inflammatory and anti–allergic effects. Quercetin is found in fruits, vegetables and grains. Onions and apples are good sources. It is also used as an ingredient in supplements.

Rutin
A plant–derived flavonoid with anti-oxidant and anti–inflammatory properties. Buckwheat is a rich dietary source of rutin.

Saturated fat
Type of food fat that is solid at room temperature. Most saturated fats come from animal food products, but some plant oils, such as palm and coconut oil, also contain high levels.

Selenium
An essential trace mineral which activates glutathione peroxidase, an antioxidant enzyme involved in the neutralisation of highly reactive molecules that contribute to aging and disease.

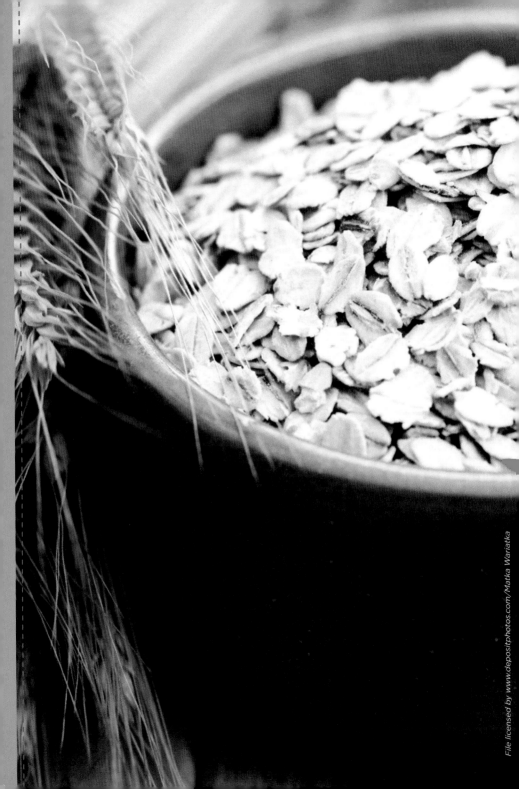

Serotonin
An important neurotransmitter (communicates information chemically between brain cells) that contributes to the regulation of sleep, appetite and mood.

Shogaol
A pungent constituent of ginger similar in chemical structure to gingerol.

Tryptophan
An amino acid that occurs in proteins, is essential for growth and normal metabolism and a precursor of niacin (vitamin B3) and serotonin.

Unsaturated fat
A fat that is liquid at room temperature and comes from plant foods. Can be monounsaturated or polyunsaturated.

Vitamin
An organic substance that plays an essential role in regulating cell functions throughout the body. Most vitamins must be obtained via diet or supplements as the body cannot produce them.

Zeaxanthin
A carotenoid found in yellow or orange plants and dark green, leafy vegetables. Zeaxanthin is being investigated for a possible association with promoting healthy vision.

REFERENCES

1. Son TG *et al* (2008) Hormetic dietary phytochemicals. *Neuromolecular Medicine* **10** (4) 236–46.

2. McCune LM *et al* (2011) Cherries and health: a review. *Critical Reviews in Food Science and Nutrition* **51** (1) 1–12.

3. Burkhardt S *et al* (2001) Detection and quantification of the anti-oxidant melatonin in Montmorency and Balaton tart cherries (Prunus Cesarus). *Journal of Agricultural and Food Chemistry* **49**, 4898–4902.

4. Wilson SJ *et al* (2010). Consensus statement on evidence-based treatment of insomnia, parasomnias and circadian rhythm disorders. *British Association for Psychopharmacology* **24** (11) 1577–601.

5. Goren-Inbar N *et al* (2002) Nuts, nut cracking, and pitted stones at Gesher Benot Ya'aqov, Israel. *Proceedings of the National Academy of Sciences* **99** (4) 2455–60.

6. Berryman CE *et al* (2011) Effects of almond consumption on the reduction of LDL-cholesterol: a discussion of potential mechanisms and future research directions. *Nutrition Reviews* **69** (4) 171–85.

7. Li SC *et al* (2011) Almond consumption improved glycemic control and lipid profiles in patients with Type 2 diabetes mellitus. *Metabolism* **60** (4) 474–9.

8. Mandalari G *et al* (2010) In vitro evaluation of the prebiotic properties of almond skins (Amygdalus communis L.). *FEMS Microbiological Letters* **304** (2) 116–22.

9. Barbosa AC *et al* (2010) Varietal influences on antihyperglycemia properties of freshly harvested apples using in vitro assay models. *Journal of Medicinal Food* **13** (6) 1313–23.

10. Mikulic Petkovsek M *et al* (2010) The influence of organic/integrated production on the content of phenolic compounds in apple leaves and fruits in four different varieties over a two-year period. *Journal of the Science of Food and Agriculture* **90** (14) 2366–78.

11. Shinohara K *et al* (2010) Effect of apple intake on fecal microbiota and metabolites in humans. *Anaerobe* **16** (5) 510–5.

12. Cassidy A *et al* (2011) Habitual intake of flavonoid subclasses and incident hypertension in adults. *American Journal of Clinical Nutrition* **93** (2) 338–47.

13. McCullough ML *et al* (2012) Flavonoid intake and cardiovascular disease mortality in a prospective cohort of US adults. American Journal of Clinical Nutrition **95** (2) 454–64.

14. Wedick NM *et al* (2012) Dietary flavonoid intakes and risk of Type 2 diabetes in US men and women. *American Journal of Clinical Nutrition* **95** (4) 925-33.

15. Malin DH *et al* (2011) Short-term blueberry-enriched diet prevents and reverses object recognition memory loss in aging rats. *Nutrition* **27** (3) 338–42.

16. Kreft I, Fabjan N and Yasumoto K (2006) Rutin content in buckwheat (Fagopyrum esculentum Moench) food materials and products. *Food Chemistry* **98** (3) 508–12.

17. Butt MS and Sultan MT (2011) Ginger and its health claims: molecular aspects. *Critical Reviews in Food Science and Nutrition* **51** (5) 383–93.

18. Kabak B and Dobson ADW (2011) An introduction to the traditional fermented foods and beverages of Turkey. *Critical Reviews in Food Science and Nutrition* **51**, 248–260.

19. Guzel-Seydim ZB *et al* (2011). Review: Functional properties of kefir. *Critical Reviews in Food Science and Nutrition* **51**, 261–268.

20. Romanin D *et al* (2010) Down-regulation of intestinal epithelial innate response by probiotic yeasts isolated from kefir. *International Journal of Food Microbiology.* **140** (2–3) 102–8.

21. Ruxton C (2010) Recommendations for the use of eggs in the diet. *Nursing Standard* **24** (37) 47–55.

22. Meydani M (2009) Potential health benefits of avenanthranides of oats. *Nutrition Reviews* **67** (12) 731–35.

23. Michele de Cuneo (1496) Letters on the second voyage, October 28, 1496. In: Samuel Eliot Morison (Ed) (1963) *Journals and other documents on the life and voyages of Christopher Columbus.* New York: Heritage Press.

24. Helms S and Miller A (2006) Natural treatment of chronic rhinosinusitis. *Alternative Medicine Review* **11** (3) 196–207.

25. Culpeper N (1653) *The Complete Herbal.* Carlisle: Applewood Books, 2006.

26. Ostman E *et al* (2005) Vinegar supplementation lowers glucose and insulin responses and increases satiety after a bread meal in healthy subjects. *European Journal of Clinical Nutrition* **59** (9) 983–88.

27. Higdon JV *et al* (2007) Cruciferous vegetables and human cancer risk: epidemiologic evidence and mechanistic basis. *Pharmacological Research* **55** (3) 224–236.

28. Ludy M and Mattes RD (2011) The effects of hedonically acceptable red pepper doses on thermogenesis and appetite. *Physiology and Behavior* **102** (3–4) 251.

29. Houston MC (2005) Nutraceuticals, vitamins, anti-oxidants, and minerals in the prevention and treatment of hypertension. *Progress in Cardiovascular Diseases* **47** (6) 396–449.

30. Yang Y *et al* (2007) Dietary chickpeas reverse visceral adiposity, dyslipidaemia and insulin resistance in rats induced by a chronic high-fat diet. *British Journal of Nutrition* **98** (4) 720–6.

31. Siebecker A (2005) Traditional bone broth in modern health and disease. *Townsend Letter*, Feb/March.

32. Rosner F *et al* (1969) *The Medical Writings of Moses Maimonides.* Philadelphia: Lippincott.

33. Rennard BO *et al.* (2000) Chicken soup inhibits neutrophil chemotaxis in vitro. *Chest* **118** (4) 1150-7.

34. Prummel W and Niekus M (2011) Late Mesolithic hunting of a small female aurochs in the valley of the River Tjonger (the Netherlands) in the light of Mesolithic aurochs hunting in NW Europe. *Journal of Archaeological Science* **38** (7) 1456-67.

35. Gislén A *et al* (2003) Superior underwater vision in a human population of sea gypsies. *Current Biology* **13** (10) 833-6.

36. Crawford MA and Broadhurst CL (2012) The role of docosahexaenoic and the marine food web as determinants of evolution and hominid brain development: the challenge for human sustainability. *Nutrition and Health* **21** (1) 17-39.

37. Tattelman E (2005) Health effects of garlic. *American Family Physician* **72** (1) 103-6.

38. Gautam S, Platel K and Srinivasan K (2010) Higher bioaccessibility of iron and zinc from food grains in the presence of garlic and onion. *Journal of Agricultural and Food Chemistry* **58** (14) 8426-8429.

39. Ramnani P *et al* (2010) Prebiotic effect of fruit and vegetable shots containing Jerusalem artichoke inulin: a human intervention study. *British Journal of Nutrition* **104** (2) 233-40.

40. Costabile A *et al* (2010) A double-blind, placebo-controlled, cross-over study to establish the bifidogenic effect of a very-long-chain inulin extracted from globe artichoke (Cynara scolymus) in healthy human subjects. *British Journal of Nutrition* **104** (7) 1007-17.

41. Yao Y *et al* (2008) Antidiabetic activity of mung bean extracts in diabetic KK-Ay mice. *Journal of Agricultural and Food Chemistry* **56** (19) 8869-73.

42. Brennan MA *et al* (2012) Amaranth, millet and buckwheat flours affect the physical properties of extruded breakfast cereals and modulates their potential glycaemic impact. *Starch - Stärke* **64** (5) 392-398.

43. Chainy GBN *et al* (2000) Anethole blocks both early and late cellular responses transduced by tumor necrosis factor: effect on NF-kB, AP-1, JNK, MAPKK and apoptosis. *Oncogene* **19** (25) 2943-50.

44. Nevin KJ and Rajamohan T (2010) Effect of topical application of virgin coconut oil on skin components and anti-oxidant status during dermal wound healing in young rats. *Skin Pharmacology and Physiology* **23** (6) 290-7.

45. Amasiri WADL and Dissanayake AS (2006) Coconut fats. *Ceylon Medical Journal* **51** (2) 47-51.

46. Pehowich DJ, Gomes AV and Barnes JA (2000) Fatty acid composition and possible health effects of coconut constituents. *West Indian Medical Journal* **49**, 128-33.

47. Nevin KG and Rajamohan T 2004) Beneficial effects of virgin coconut oil on lipid parameters and in vitro LDL oxidation. *Clinical Biochemistry* **37**, 830-5.

48. Bergsson G, Steingrimsson O and Thormar H (2002) Bactericidal effects of fatty acids and monoglycerides on Helicobacter pylori. *International Journal of Antimicrobial Agents* **20**, 258–62.

49. Ghanbari R *et al* (2012) Valuable nutrients and functional bioactives in different parts of olive (Olea europaea L.) – a review. *International Journal of Molecular Sciences* **13** (3) 3291–340.

50. Mafuvadze B *et al* (2011) Apigenin prevents development of medroxyprogesterone acetate-accelerated 7,12-dimethylbenz(a) anthracene-induced mammary tumors in Sprague–Dawley rats. *Cancer Prevention Research* (Phila) **4** (8) 1316–24.

51. Revedin A *et al* (2010) Thirty thousand-year-old evidence of plant food processing. *Proceedings of the National Academy of Sciences USA* **107** (44) 18815–9.

52. Artisan Bread Organic at www.artisanbread–abo.com

53. Vega-Gálvez A *et al* (2010) Nutrition facts and functional potential of quinoa (Chenopodium quinoa willd.), an ancient Andean grain: a review. *Journal of Science and Food Agriculture* **90** (15) 2541–7.

54. Pathak DR *et al* (2005) Joint association of high cabbage/sauerkraut intake at 12–13 years of age and adulthood with reduced breast cancer risk in Polish migrant women: results from the US component of the Polish women's health study. Abstract number 3697. Presented at the *AACR 4th Annual Conference on Frontiers in Cancer Prevention Research*, October 30–November 2, Baltimore, Maryland.

55. Klarin B *et al* (2008) Use of the probiotic Lactobacillus plantarum 299 to reduce pathogenic bacteria in the oropharynx of intubated patients: a randomised controlled open pilot study. *Critical Care* **12**, R136.

56. Hernández A *et al* (2012) Dietary nitrate increases tetanic [Ca2+]i and contractile force in mouse fast–twitch muscle. *Journal of Physiology* **590** (Pt 15), 3575–83.

57. Georg Lietz *et al* (2009) Two common single nucleotide polymorphisms in the gene encoding beta-carotene 15,15%u2019-monoxygenase alter beta-carotene metabolism in female volunteers. *The FASEB Journal* **23**,1041–1053.

58. Bahado-Singh PS *et al* (2011) Relationship between processing method and the glycemic indices of ten sweet potato (ipomoea batatas) cultivars commonly consumed in Jamaica. *Journal of Nutrition and Metabolism* Article ID 584832, doi:10.1155/2011/584832.

59. Ben Johnson (1298) *The Travels of Marco Polo: The Venetian*, as translated and republished in 2010 in Whitefish, MT, USA by Kessinger Publishing.

60. Chandran B and Goel A (2012) A randomized, pilot study to assess the efficacy and safety of curcumin in patients with active rheumatoid arthritis. *Phytotherapy Research*, March 9, Epublished ahead of print.

61. Sikora E, Scapagnini G and Barbagallo M (2010) Curcumin, inflammation, ageing and age-related diseases. *Immunity & Aging* **7** (1) 1.

62. Cowan AK and Wolstenholme BN (2003) Avocados. In: *Encyclopedia of Food Sciences and Nutrition (Second Edition)*, pp348–353.

63. Lopez Ledesma R *et al* (1996) Monounsaturated fatty acid (avocado) rich diet for mild hypercholesterolemia. *Archives of Medical Research* **27** (4) 519–523.

64. Wootton-Beard PC and Ryan L (2011) A beetroot juice shot is a significant and convenient source of bioaccessible anti-oxidants. *Journal of Functional Foods* **3** (4) 329–34.

65. Hobbs DA *et al* (2012) Blood pressure-lowering effects of beetroot juice and novel beetroot-enriched bread products in normotensive male subjects. *British Journal of Nutrition* **108**, (11) 2066–74.

66. Hooper L *et al* (2012) Effects of chocolate, cocoa, and flavan-3-ols on cardiovascular health: a systematic review and meta-analysis of randomized trials. *American Journal of Clinical Nutrition* **95** (3) 740–51.

67. http://www.ars.usda.gov/research/docs.htm?docid=8877 sourced online 2.1.2012

68. Qin B, Panickar KS and Anderson RA (2010) Cinnamon: Potential role in the prevention of insulin resistance, metabolic syndrome, and type 2 diabetes. *Journal of Diabetes Scientific Technology* **4** (3) 685–693.

69. Frequently Asked Questions about coumarin in cinnamon and other foods, The Federal Institute for Risk Assessment (BfR) (sourced online on 31.12.11 at http://www.bfr.bund.de/en/frequently_asked_questions_about_coumarin_in_cinnamon_and_other_foods–8487.html

70. Rafehi H, Ververis K and Karagiannis TC (2011) Controversies surrounding the clinical potential of cinnamon for the management of diabetes. *Diabetes, Obesity & Metabolism* **14** (6) 493–9.

71. Smoliga JM, Baur JA and Hausenblas HA (2011) Resveratrol and health – a comprehensive review of human clinical trials. *Molecular Nutrition and Food Research* **55**, 1129–1141.

72. Al-Waili N, Salom K and Al-Ghamdi AA (2011) Honey for wound healing, ulcers, and burns; data supporting its use in clinical practice. *Scientific World Journal* **11**, 766–87.

73. Breeze TD, Roberts SPM and Potts SG (2012) *The Decline of England's Bees: Policy review and recommendations*. Reading: University of Reading.

74. Ejike EC and Ezeanyika LU (2011) Inhibition of the experimental induction of benign prostatic hyperplasia: a possible role for fluted pumpkin (Telfairia occidentalis Hook f.) seeds. *Urologia Internationalis* **87** (2) 218–24.

75. Callaway J *et al* (2005) Efficacy of dietary hempseed oil in patients with atopic dermatitis. *Journal of Dermatological Treatment* **16** (2) 87–94.

76. Singh KK *et al* (2011) Flaxseed: a potential source of food, feed and fiber. *Critical Reviews in Food Science and Nutrition* **51** (3) 210–222.

77. Thakorlal J *et al* (2010) Resistant starch in Micronesian banana cultivars offers health benefits. P*acific Health Dialogue* **16** (1) 49–59.

USEFUL RESOURCES

Books

Fallon S (2001)
Nourishing Traditions
(2nd edition). Washington DC:
New Trends Publishing.

Campbell-McBride N (2004)
Gut and Psychology Syndrome: Natural Treatment for Autism, ADD/ADHD, Dyslexia, Dyspraxia, Depression, Schizophrenia
(2nd Revised edition). Medinform Publishing.

Campbell-McBride N (2007)
Put Your Heart in Your Mouth.
Medinform Publishing.

Nicolle L and Bailey C (2012)
The Functional Nutrition Cookbook.
London: Singing Dragon.

Katz SE (2003) *Wild Fermentation: the flavor, nutrition, and craft of live-culture foods.*
Chelsea Green Publishing Co, US.

Watts M (Ed) (2008)
Nutrition and Mental Health: A handbook.
Brighton: Pavilion Publishing Ltd.

Watts M (Ed) (2011)
Nutrition and Addiction: A handbook.
Brighton: Pavilion Publishing Ltd.

Websites

http://www.foodsmatter.com
A resource for allergy, intolerance and sensitivity.

http://www.fabresearch.org
Food and Behaviour Research is a charitable organisation dedicated both to advancing scientific research into the links between nutrition and human behaviour and to making these findings available to the widest possible audience.

http://www.functionalmedicine.org
Functional medicine addresses the underlying causes of disease, using a systems-oriented approach and engaging both patient and practitioner in a therapeutic partnership.

http://www.mccarrisonsociety.org.uk
The McCarrison Society for Nutrition and Health is a charitable organisation assembling scientific knowledge on nutrition and health free from economic and political pressures, to help secure the physical and mental health of future generations.

http://www.bant.org.uk
The British Association for Applied Nutrition and Nutritional Therapy (BANT) is the professional body for Nutritional Therapists.

NOTES

NOTES

NOTES

NOTES

Other titles in the *49 Ways to Well-being Series* include:

49 Ways to Think Yourself Well
49 Ways to Write Yourself Well
49 Ways to Move Yourself Well
49 Ways to Mental Health Recovery
49 Ways to Sexual Well-being

For more details visit
www.stepbeachpress.co.uk/well-being